HEALTHY DESSERT COOKBOOK

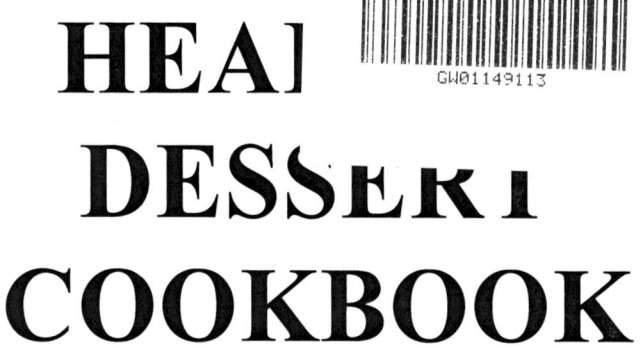

SUGAR-FREE AND GLUTEN-FREE HEALTHY RECIPES DESSERT COOKBOOK

DIANA POLSKA

Copyright © 2016

All rights reserved. No part of this book may be reproduced or transmitted in any form or by any electronic or mechanical means, including photocopy, recording, or any information storage and retrieval system now known or to be invented, without written permission from the author, except by a reviewer who wishes to quote brief passages in connection with a review written for inclusion in a magazine, newspaper, website, or broadcast.

Disclaimer: Neither the author nor the publisher shall be held liable or responsible to any person or entity with respect to any loss or incidental or consequential damages caused, directly or indirectly, by the information or programs contained herein. You must seek the services of a competent professional before beginning any health or weight-loss advice. References are provided for informational purposes only. They do not constitute endorsement of any websites or other sources.

CONTENTS

INTRODUCTION..7
- HEALTHY DESSERT INGREDIENTS......................7
- UNHEALTHY SWEETENERS..................................8
- HEALTHY SWEETENERS.....................................10

RECIPES...13
- NUTTY PEACH AND PEAR BARS 14
- HEALTHY FRUIT POPSICLES 17
- CUTE FRUIT BITES..19
- ALMOND BUTTER SNACKS.................................21
- PEACH MELBA 23
- SUGARLESS PEACH COBBLER 25
- NUTRITIVE COOKIES..27
- ANYTIME ENERGY BARS 29
- BANANA FUN TREATS 31
- STRAWBERRY MOUSSE 33
- PERFECTLY ACCEPTABLE BROWNIES 35
- LEMON DELIGHT 37
- YOU NEW FAVORITE CHOCOLATE COOKIES ...40
- DARKER ANGEL FOOD CAKE 42
- PEACH AND STRAWBERRIES SHAKE 44
- CHOCOLATE AND COFFEE MERINGUES 46
- BREAKFAST OR DESSERT SMOOTHIE...............48
- GREEN BUT SWEET SMOOTHIE IDEA...............50
- CHEESE AND PEARS DELICIOUS COMBO 52
- ZUCCHINI CHOCOLATE BREAD 54
- BANANA FRENCH TOASTS EGGS FREE............56
- CHOCOLATE AND CHERRIES LOW CARBS CAKE 58
- THE PERFECT LOW SUGARS FLAN 61
- NO FLOUR VANILLA AND ALMOND CAKE.......63
- CHOCOLATE COOKIES WITH PEPPERMINT SPLASH........65

A SIMPLY DELICIOUS PINEAPPLE CAKE	67
A CHOCOLATE BREAD DELIGHT IDEA	69
CRANBERRY PINEAPPLE BREAD PUDDING	71
THE PERFECT CAKE DUO: CHOCOLATE AND PUMPKIN	73
MANGO CREPES	75
SUGARCANE FLAVORED CUSTARD	77
CHOCOLATE CREPES WITH FRUITS	79
DELECTABLE PEANUT COOKIES	81
SWEET TEA FOR DESSERT	83
CUPCAKES FROM THE ISLANDS	85
SUPER CLASSIC BREAD PUDDING	87
SOUR CREAM AND NUTS CAKE	89
CHERRY DELIGHT	91
PEANUT BUTTER BROWNIES	93
THE ALMOST TOO GOOD TO BE TRUE DESSERT	96
DELICIOUS BERRIES SQUARE	98
HERBS AND MELON FROZEN TREATS	100
STRAWBERRY AND CHEESE LOG	102
SIMPLE BANANA BREAD	105
EVERYDAY MUFFINS	107
SPICY CARROT BITES	109
DRESSED UP PEACHES	111
CARROT MUFFINS FOR EVERYONE	113
UNIQUE RASPBERRY SOUP	115
WHO WANTS SUSHI?	117
RASPBERRIES AND POPPY SEEDS MUFFINS	119
DELICIOUS DIP FOR YOUR FAVORITE FRUITS	121
SWEET POTATOES CASSEROLE	123
DRIED CRANBERRIES AND WALNUTS SCONES	126
BANANA AND ALMOND BUTTER SMOOTHIE	128
CRISPY BREAKFAST	130
YOGOURT DIP	132
THE SMOOTHIEST PIE	134
DRIED FRUITS AND NUTS YUMMY SQUARES	136
VANILLA WARM BEVERAGE	138
MELON SALAD	140
GINGERBREAD TASTY LOAF	142

- MY FAVORITE PEANUT BUTTER COOKIES..................145
- A LITTLE SOMETHING TO TOP OFF A FRUIT SALAD......147
- APPLE AND RAISINS TOPPING..........................149
- FUN POPSICLES 151
- VERY BERRIES SMOOTHIE..............................153
- YOUR KID'S LUNCH BOX 155
- APPLE CRUMBLES FOR EVERYONE 158
- DELICIOUS ANYTIME BITES 160
- MIXED APPLE SAUCE 162
- "BLUE" GRANITA 164
- ORANGE MUFFINS.....................................166
- NOT ANOTHER GREEN SMOOTHIE 169
- BAKED APPLES......................................171
- TOO GOOD TO BE TRUE CANDIES 173
- THE PERFECT HOLIDAY LOAF 175
- PEAR AND HONEY SCONES 177
- ANOTHER INTERESTING BROWNIES RECIPE 179
- SWEET POTATO PIE, JUST SWEET ENOUGH................181
- DID YOU SAY HEALTHY DONUTS? 183
- DIABETIC APPROVED PUMPKIN PIE 186
- DATES BREAD.......................................188
- ZUCHINNI CITRUS BREAD 190
- MUFFINS FILLED WITH PEACHES........................192
- PEANUT BUTTER DELIGHT 194
- SCOTTISH LIKE SCONES...............................196
- FRUITS SKEWERS 198
- ORANGE APPLE CLAFOUTI 200
- REINVENTEED ANGEL FOOD CAKE 202
- CUTE ELEPHANT EARS 205
- YOUR DIABETIC EGGNOG VERSION.......................208
- STRAWBERRY PARFAIT 210
- DELICIOUS BANANA AND MORE COOKIES 212
- A DIABETIC GREEN TEA SMOOTHIE......................215
- SOME BALLS OF GOODNESS 217
- YUMMY SANDWICH COOKIES.............................219
- THIS MAGESTIC BANANAS AND BERRIES TREAT 221
- CHOCO-CHEESE NO BAKE PIE...........................223

CHOCOLATE MINTY PUDDING 225
AVOCADO AND PEANUT BUTTER SHAKE 227
PINEAPPLE SIMPLE BARS 229

INTRODUCTION

You can eat dessert and still be lean and healthy. Using natural sweeteners instead of sugar to sweeten all desserts is such a simple way to reduce weight gain caused by the excessive consumption of sweets.

If every bakery, cake maker, chocolate maker, and candy manufacturer used stevia or other low glycemic index natural sweeteners instead of sugar, then obesity would not be such a crushing problem. Dieting or dietary restrictions would not be necessary, and you could eat dessert at each meal if you really had a desire for it.

HEALTHY DESSERT INGREDIENTS

For cookies, cupcakes, donuts, muffins, pancakes, waffles, brownies, cakes, pies, and all other desserts and baked goods, you can substitute a few ingredients to make these desserts healthier and lower in calorie density. The two main ingredients to eliminate are white flour and white sugar, as both have high glycemic values, causing blood sugar control problems and weight gain.

You can replace wheat flour with coconut flour, quinoa flour, oat flour, spelt flour, kamut flour, rye flour, barley flour, or buckwheat flour. Coconut flour is a popular choice. It is high in fiber, low on the GI, and gluten-free. Oat flour is another popular choice. It tastes a lot like white flour but is much healthier. It's lower on the GI and is a rich source of soluble fiber.

You can replace white sugar with low GI, natural sweeteners such as pure stevia, coconut palm sugar, sugarcane juice, Manuka honey, and sweet proteins (Brazzein, Thaumatin, Monelin, Curculin, Mabinlin, Miraculin, Pentadin). Not everyone reacts to these sugars the same way, even if they are low in the GI, so it's best to buy a glucose meter and test your blood sugar before and after eating one of these sweeteners to see which works best for you.

UNHEALTHY SWEETENERS

There are so many disadvantages of eating sugar. High sugar intake increases advanced glycation end products (AGEs), which are sugar molecules that attach to and damage proteins in the body. AGEs speed up the aging of cells, which may contribute to a variety of chronic and fatal diseases.

Sugar produces a rise in triglycerides, a leading cause of heart disease. Sugar feeds cancer cells and has been connected to the development of cancer of the breast, ovaries, prostate, rectum, pancreas, biliary tract, lung, gallbladder, and stomach. Sugar can also cause arthritis, multiple sclerosis, diabetes, osteoporosis, Alzheimer's disease, cataracts, kidney damage, and adrenal gland dysfunction.

Agave syrup has become popular in recent years, but it's not a good choice. The Glycemic Research Institute announced that it has stopped all future clinical trials of agave as a result of the latest clinical trials, in which diabetic subjects experienced severe and dangerous side effects related to the consumption of agave. The institute also legally de-listed and placed a ban on agave for use in foods, beverages, chocolate, and other products. Manufacturers that produce and use agave in products are warned that they can be held legally liable for negative health incidents related to ingestion of agave.

Artificial sweeteners are not recommended. They have been linked to increased cancer risk. Long-term use of artificial sweeteners has been linked to headaches, seizures, blindness, and cognitive and behavioral changes.

Artificial sweeteners such as saccharin (Sugar Twin, Sweet 'N Low), aspartame (Equal, NutraSweet), sucralose (Splenda), acesulfame potassium (also known as acesulfame k—Sunett, Sweet One), neotame, and tagatose are linked to a number of health problems. Numerous studies show that frequent consumption of low-calorie artificial sweeteners causes weight gain and increases one's risk for metabolic syndrome, type 2 diabetes, and cardiovascular disease.

The consumption of artificial sweeteners leads to increased body weight and obesity because it interferes with the normal functions of the body. In one study, consumption of artificial sweeteners increased BMI and increased body fat percentage at a two-year follow-up.

Even though low-calorie artificial sweeteners are currently approved for use, many people have reported that they believe their negative health symptoms were caused by these artificial sugar substitutes.

HEALTHY SWEETENERS

Coconut palm sugar, stevia, and raw organic Manuka honey are the best natural sweeteners to use and even have some health benefits.

Coconut palm sugar is a very good sugar substitute. It is low on the GI (with a GI of 35), and rich in potassium, magnesium, zinc, iron, and B vitamins.

Stevia has been widely used for centuries in South America as well as in Japan. It has zero calories and has a GI of zero, which means it does not raise blood sugar levels. Unlike sugar, which has a negative effect on those with diabetes, stevia has been shown to have a positive effect on those with diabetes. Studies have found that stevia improves insulin sensitivity, promotes additional insulin production, and helps reverse diabetes and metabolic syndrome.

The medicinal use of products made by honeybees is called apitherapy. The use of honey and propolis in the treatment and prevention of numerous diseases has been documented. Honey has demonstrated bactericidal activity against salmonella, Shigella, Escherichia coli, and H. pylori.

Research demonstrates that propolis has the highest antioxidant power, followed by royal jelly and honey. Propolis has antibacterial, antifungal, antiviral, antioxidative, antiparasitic, immunomodulating, anti-inflammatory, analgesic, hepatoprotective, and anti-carcinogenic effects. Royal jelly has antitumor effects.

The antibacterial activity in Manuka honey is much stronger than in other types of honey. "UMF" stands for "Unique Manuka Factor" and is a property that gives Manuka honey its special healing quality. UMF Manuka honey with a rating of 16+ has the highest level of antibacterial activity. Manuka honey is best consumed raw, as heat destroys the nutrients in honey.

Lo han guo is an exotic fruit extract that has zero calories and zero glycemic impact, making it safe for diabetics and hypoglycemics to use. Lo han guo can be used in your baking as a sugar substitute.

Xylitol is just as sweet as table sugar (sucrose) but has about 40 percent fewer calories and 75 percent fewer carbohydrates. Xylitol also won't raise your blood sugar like regular sugar does, as the body does not require insulin to metabolize xylitol.

Raw honey is a good sugar substitute, has a low glycemic response, and is suitable for those with diabetes. Raw, unprocessed honey has antioxidants, minerals, vitamins, amino acids, enzymes, and phytonutrients. It is considered a superfood. It is good for sweetening tea, coffee, or drinks. Pasteurized honey has a higher GI, so always use raw, unheated honey.

Coconut palm sugar has a lower GI (35) than does white sugar. It is rich in magnesium, potassium, zinc, and B vitamins. In terms of taste, out of all the natural sweeteners, it comes closest to white sugar. It's good for baking and sweetening coffee, tea, or smoothies.

Raw sugarcane juice has a low GI. It has no simple sugars and doesn't cause blood sugar to soar like white sugar does. It contains calcium, magnesium, potassium, iron, and manganese.

Lucuma powder is made from whole Peruvian lucuma fruit. It is rich in minerals such as iron, zinc, potassium, calcium, magnesium, vitamin B3, and beta carotene. Lucuma has a low GI and GL.

Stevia comes in powdered or liquid form. It's a good substitute for white sugar when baking. Stevia is sweeter than sugar, so you need less of it. It has no effect on blood sugar levels. It has a GI of zero, and it has zero calories.

Sweet proteins (Brazzein, Thaumatin, Monelin, Curculin, Mabinlin, Miraculin, Pentadin) have been isolated from plants that grow in tropical rainforests. Sweet proteins are thousands of times sweeter than sucrose. They are of low calorie value, and can safely be used as sweeteners by people suffering from diseases linked to consumption of sugar e.g. obesity, diabetes and hyperlipemia.

RECIPES

NUTTY PEACH AND PEAR BARS

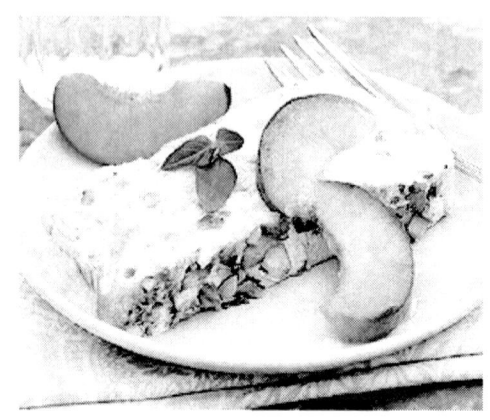

Makes:
8-10 Servings

Preparation time:
20 minutes

Ingredients:
2 ripe fresh pear (pitted and sliced) –save one for garnish
3 ripe fresh peach (cored and sliced)- save one sliced peach for garnish
¼ cup pistachios
¼ cup walnuts
2 Tbsp. lime juice
3 eggs
1 cup coconut cream
¼ cup coconut sugar
½ tsp. salt
½ tsp. vanilla extract
Coconut oil (to grease pan)

Directions:

1. Grease a square baking dish with coconut oil first.
2. In the food processor, you should then place 2 of the peaches (chunks), 1 one of the pear (chunks), the lime juice, and 3 Tbsp. of coconut sugar.
3. Once it has become a puree, set it aside.
4. In a mixing bowl, combine the eggs, salt and the rest of the coconut sugar. Whisk well.
5. Then, in a saucepan, boil some water and place the bowl with eggs mixture over the boiling water for just 3 or 4 minutes. This should allow the mixture to become your filling (texture similar to a pudding). Set aside and let it cool off after for 10 minutes.
6. Next, mix together the fruit's mixture and vanilla extract.
7. Add also the eggs mixture to the puree. Finally add the walnuts and pistachios to the mixture.
8. Pour the delicious fruity mixture into the dish and cover it with plastic wrap.
9. You should refrigerate for at least 12 hours, overnight works well.
10. When serving, use the fresh sliced peach and pear to decorate if you like and you could also sprinkle with coconut sugar if you like.

11. Cut the bars the size you like and enjoy with a nice cup of tea.

Nutrition Information per serving: 169 Calories, 7 g total fat, 60 mg cholesterol, 36 mg sodium, **22 g carbonates (sugars),** 2.1g fiber, and 4g protein.

HEALTHY FRUIT POPSICLES

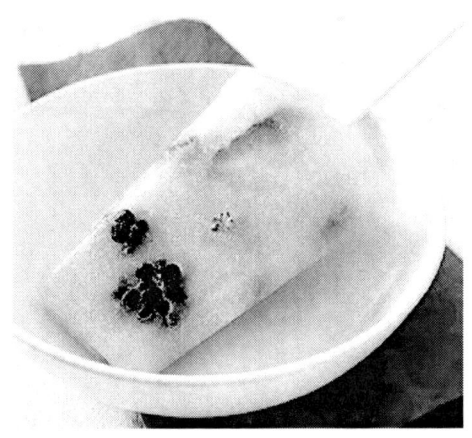

Makes:
16-24 Servings

Preparation time:
5 minutes

Ingredients:
1 large jar unsweetened apple sauce (your favorite brand)
1 Tsp. lemon juice
Pinch ground cinnamon
1 cup fresh blueberries
1 cup fresh blackberries

Directions:

1. Wash the berries and set them aside.

2. In a large bowl, combine the applesauce, the lemon juice, the cinnamon and the fruits. Pour the mixture into Popsicle molds.

3. You could also use some ice trays and stick Popsicle sticks (cut in halves if needed) in them.

4. Place in the freezer for at least 12 hours (overnight).

5. Lick away!

Nutrition Information per serving: 39 Calories, 7.5 g total fat, 0 mg cholesterol, 1 mg sodium, **8.5 g carbonates (sugars),** 1g fiber, and 0.5g protein.

CUTE FRUIT BITES

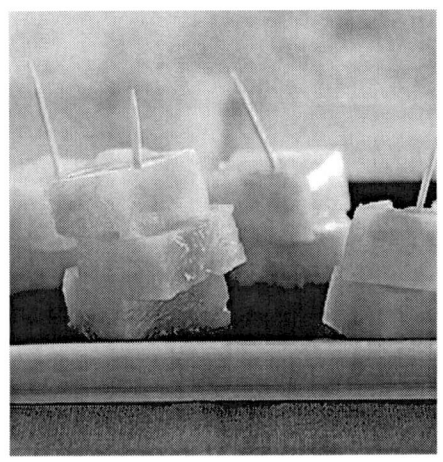

Makes:
12-14 Servings

Preparation time:
30 minutes

Ingredients:
2 cups pineapple juice
1 cup orange juice
1 cup mango juice
3 envelopes unflavored gelatin (dry)
1 cup small pineapple chunks

Directions:

1. In a bowl you should toss the gelatin powder over the orange, mango and pineapple juices.

2. If needed, add a little hot water to help the gelatin dissolve.

3. Next pour this mixture into a square baking dish.

4. Place the dish in the freezer for about 40 minutes.

5. When you remove it, add the pineapple chunks.

6. Keep in the refrigerator until ready to serve and cut in small or big squares!

7. Kids and adults will love these!

Nutrition Information per serving: 130 Calories, 0.2 g total fat, 0 mg cholesterol, 31 mg sodium, **22.2 g carbonates (sugars),** 1.2.g fiber, and 2g protein.

ALMOND BUTTER SNACKS

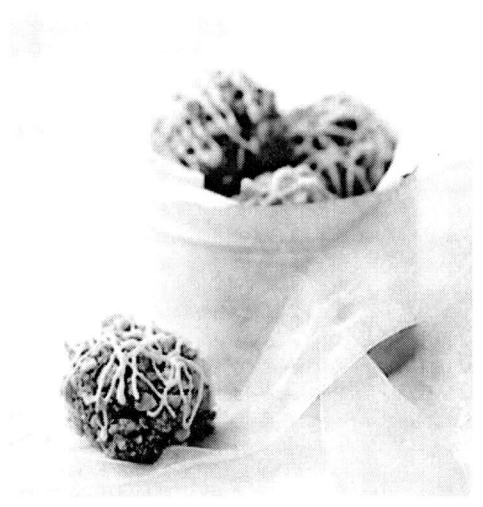

Makes:
18-20 Servings

Preparation time:
15 minutes

Ingredients:
1/3 cup almond butter
¼ cup coconut oil
1/cup raw Manuka honey
1 cup coconut flour
¼ cup unsweetened coconut flakes
¼ cup flaxseeds
¼ cup chopped almonds
½ tsp. ground nutmeg

Directions:

1. In a medium pot, mix the almond butter, coconut oil and honey and bring to boil.

2. Remove from heat; add the rest of the ingredients.

3. Transfer the mixture into a mixing bowl, and let the mixture cool off for 5 minutes.

4. Then use your hands to prepare the balls.

5. Adjust coconut flour or coconut oil, if you are not satisfied with the texture.

6. Refrigerate these small almond snacks in a plastic container.

Nutrition Information per serving: 103 Calories, 5.5 g total fat, 1.2 mg cholesterol, 68 mg sodium, **11.1 g carbonates (sugars),** 2.1g fiber, and 2g protein.

PEACH MELBA

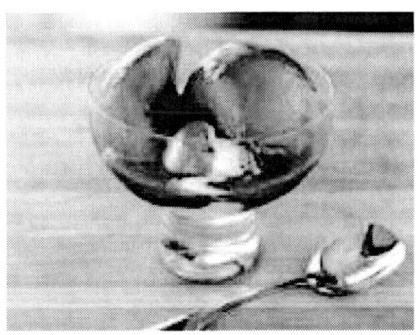

Makes:
6 Servings

Prep:
10 minutes

Ingredients:
1 Tbsp. raspberry naturally favored tea mix (make sure it's low calories and sugar free)
1 Tbsp. peach naturally favored tea mix (make sure it's low calories and sugar free)
1 cup cold water
1 small package sugar free raspberry flavored gelatin
1 small package sugar free raspberry flavored gelatin
2 Cups boiling water
1 cup sliced peaches (frozen or canned are okay, just make sure they are sugar free as well)
Coconut cream if desired

Directions:

1. In a medium size bowl, dissolve both tea mixes, with some cold water.

2. Secondly, it's time to dissolve the gelatin in a different mixing bowl by pouring the hot water on it.

3. Add the tea mixture to the gelatin mixture and refrigerate.

4. After about an hour, you should be left with a mixture that is somewhat firm.

5. Using your favorite serving cups, pour the 1 cup of gelatin mix, add some peaches and some coconut cream (to taste).

6. Make sure to refrigerate until ready to serve (it should be cooled down at least 4-5 hours before it will be ready to eat).

Nutrition Information per serving: 35 Calories, 5.5 g total fat, 1.2 mg cholesterol, 38 mg sodium, **5.1 g carbonates (sugars),** 1.9g fiber, and 1g protein.

SUGARLESS PEACH COBBLER

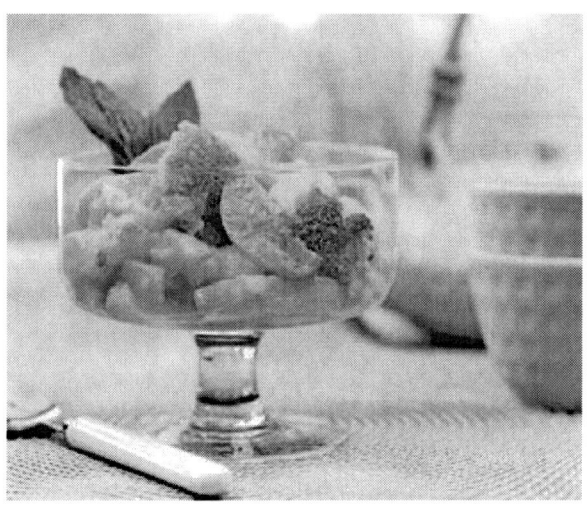

Makes:
6 Servings

Preparation time:
35 minutes

Ingredients:
Filling
1 large can no sugar added peaches (save the juice)
2 Tsp. raw organic Manuka honey
Pinch ground cinnamon
2 Tbsp. coconut toil (room temperature)
Crust(topping)
5 Tbsp. oat flour
1/4 cup coconut oil (room temperature)
4 Tbsp. coconut palm sugar
Pinch salt
Some water

Directions:

1. Preheat the oven to 325 degrees F.

2. Prepare a large baking by greasing it with a little coconut oil.

3. For the filling, simply mix all the ingredients together, except the peaches.

4. Place the peaches on the bottom of the dish and pour the mixture on top.

5. For the topping, mix the ingredients in a separate bowl first and add some water to get the wanted consistency. It should be crumbly.

6. Finally sprinkle the crust on top of the peaches.

7. Bake in the oven for about 30 minutes or so.

Nutrition Information per serving: 290 Calories, 24.5 g total fat, 0 mg cholesterol, 108 mg sodium, **21.5 g carbonates (sugars),** 13g fiber, and 1.5g protein.

NUTRITIVE COOKIES

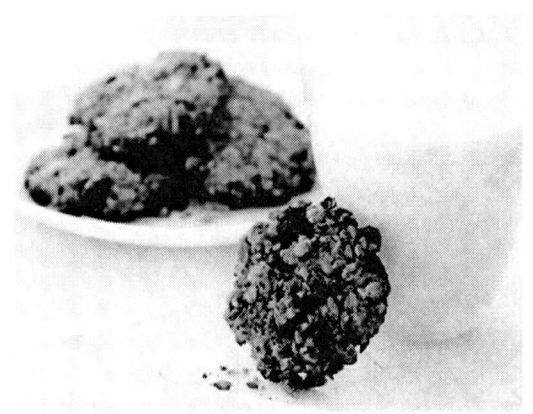

Makes:
16-20 Servings

Preparation time:
15 minutes

Ingredients:
2 Tbsp. finale chopped walnuts
1 Tbsp. finale chopped sunflower seeds
½ cup finally chopped dried dates
1 Tbsp. pure Stevia
1 cup almond flour
½ tsp. baking soda
2 Tbsp. coconut oil (room temperature)
4 Tbsp. unsweetened apple juice

Directions:

1. Preheat the oven to 325 degrees F.

2. In a food processor, place the walnuts, sunflowers and dates, activate a few times. It will be a little pasty.

3. Place next that mixture of nuts and dates in a large mixing bowl, add the almond flour, the baking soda, Stevia and stir well.

4. Add to the mixture the coconut oil now and the apple juice. Stir again and your cookie dough should be ready to bake.

5. On a greased baking sheet drop the cookie dough (about a teaspoon each), spacing it out at least an inch between.

6. Bake in the oven for about 10 minutes.

7. Let the cookies cool down before you store them a container for storage.

Nutrition Information per serving: 69 Calories, 3 g total fat, 0 mg cholesterol, 41 mg sodium, **9 g carbonates (sugars),** 1 g fiber, and 1g protein.

ANYTIME ENERGY BARS

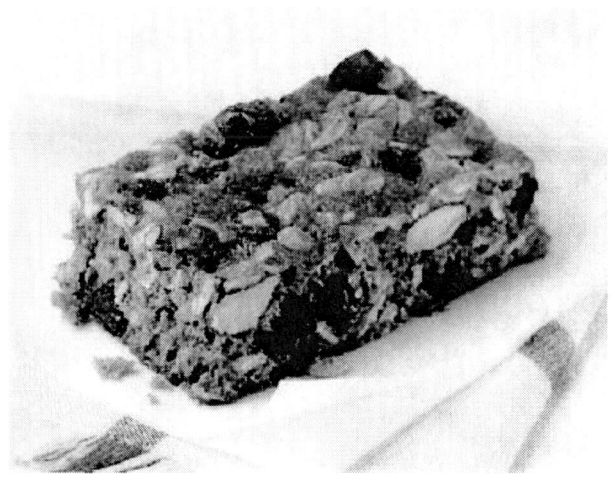

Makes:
24 Servings

Preparation time:
45 minutes

Ingredients:
2 cups quinoa flour
¼ cup flaxseeds
1/2 tsp. baking soda
Pinch salt
1 tsp. ground cinnamon
3/4 cup natural-(unsweetened) smooth peanut butter
½ cup Manuka honey
2 large eggs
2 Tbsp. walnut oil
3/4 cup dried cherries
3/4 cup chopped almonds

Directions:

1. Preheat the oven to 350 degrees F.

2. Grease a rectangle baking dish with a little coconut oil or non-tick cooking spray.

3. In a large mixing bowl, combine the first 5 ingredients.

4. In a different bowl, mix the peanut butter, eggs and honey.

5. Combine the 2 mixtures together and stir well.

6. Finally add the dried cherries and almonds. Mix again.

7. Pour the mixture in the baking dish. Bake in the oven for about 25 minutes.

8. Let it cool off before you start cutting.

Nutrition Information per serving: 172 Calories, 7.9 g total fat, 10 mg cholesterol, 68 mg sodium, **23 g carbonates (sugars),** 2g fiber, and 4g protein.

BANANA FUN TREATS

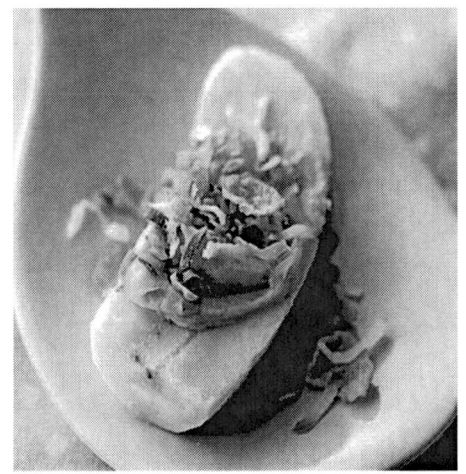

Makes:
4 Servings

Preparation time:
5 minutes

Ingredients:
2 Tbsp. shredded coconut
2 Tbsp. low fat no sugar added yoghurt
2 Tbsp. almond butter
2 bananas

Directions:

1. You can choose to roast the shredded coconut or not. If you choose too, the easiest way it sot heat it up for a few minutes in coconut oil in a skillet.

2. Prepare the bananas by slicing them in half.

3. In a bowl, mix the yogurt, almond butter. Spread on each banana piece and sprinkle some shredded coconut on top.

Nutrition Information per serving: 69 Calories, 2 g total fat, 60 mg cholesterol, 32 mg sodium, **11 g carbonates (sugars),** 1.1g fiber, and 3g protein.

STRAWBERRY MOUSSE

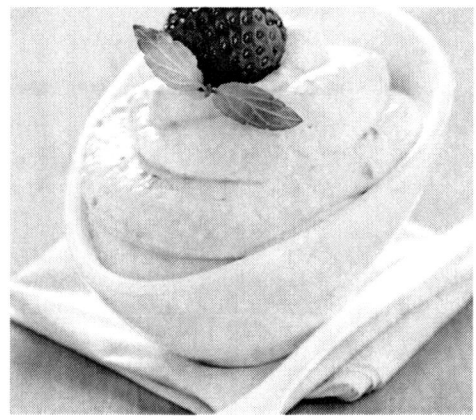

Makes:
8-10 Servings

Preparation time:
20 minutes

Ingredients:

1 X 8 ounces package low fat cream cheese (room temperature)
1 cup unsweetened coconut milk (divided)
3 Tbsp. strawberry natural flavoring (natural drink mix, exclude any drink mix with artificial sweeteners)

Directions:

1. Beat the cream cheese in a medium mixing bowl, and start by adding half of the required strawberry flavoring mix. I highly suggest using an electric

mixer so it is easier to get to the wanted consistency.

2. Alternate adding the coconut milk and the rest of the strawberry mix to the first mixture and continue mixing.

3. You should refrigerate your mousse for about 3 hours before serving.

4. I like to serve this dessert in fancy cups!

Nutrition Information per serving: 85 Calories, 3 g total fat, 3 mg cholesterol, 130 mg sodium, **9 g carbonates (sugars),** 0g fiber, and 5g protein.

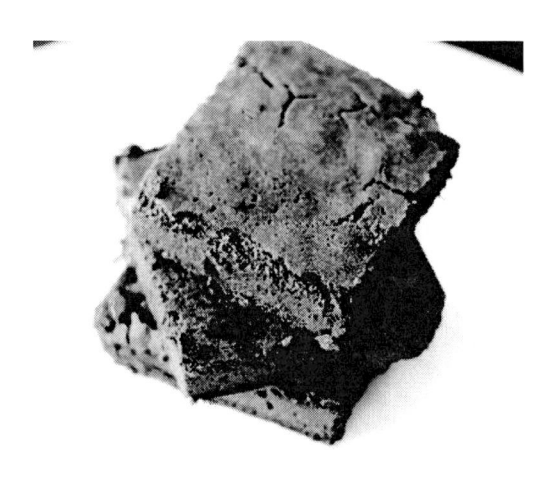

PERFECTLY ACCEPTABLE BROWNIES

Makes:
12-16 Servings

Preparation time:
1 hour

Ingredients:
1 cup unsalted grass fed butter
2 Tbsp. unsweetened cashew milk
1 ½ coconut palm sugar
5 large eggs
1 tsp. pure vanilla
8 Tbsp. unsweetened cocoa powder

Directions

1. Preheat oven to 350 degrees F.

2. In a small saucepan, heat on low the butter, the cashew milk and the cocoa powder. Whisk so no lumps form.

3. In a bowl, mix the eggs and the coconut palm sugar.

4. Next pour slowly the chocolate mixture, and stir constantly.

5. In a greased square pan, pour the mixture and bake for about 45 to 50 minutes.

6. These brownies will be fluffy. Let them cool down before you start cutting them in squares.

Nutrition Information per serving: 55 Calories, 50 g total fat, 44 mg cholesterol, 10 mg sodium, **3 g carbonates (sugars),** 1g fiber, and 7g protein.

LEMON DELIGHT

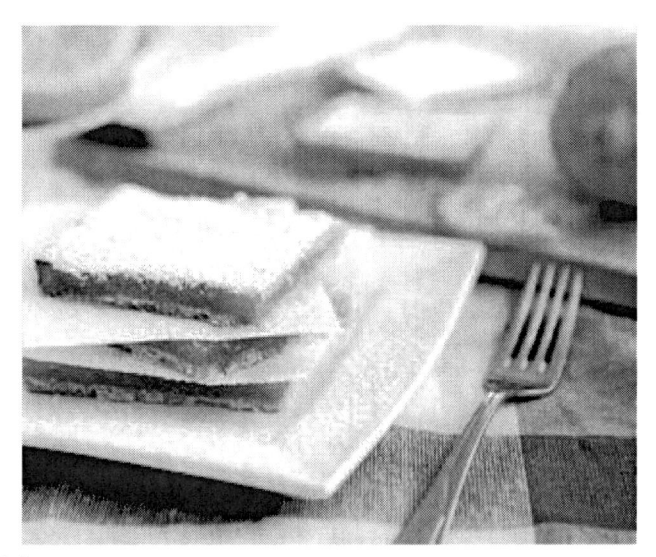

Makes:
10-12 Servings

Preparation time:
35 minutes

Ingredients:
Crust
1 cup quinoa flour
Pinch salt
2 Tbsp. coconut palm sugar
1 Tbsp. coconut oil (room temperature)
2 Tbsp. grass fed butter
1 Tbsp. sugar cane juice
Filling
1/4 cup coconut flour (fine ground)
½ cup. Coconut plan sugar

2 Tbps. Manuka honey

5 medium eggs

1/2 cup lemon juice

Directions

1. Preheat oven to 350 degrees F. With some coconut oil, lightly grease a square or rectangle baking dish.

2. Prepare the crust first by combining the quinoa flour, salt and coconut palm sugar.

3. In a different bowl, mix the coconut oil, butter and sugar cane juice. Mix well. The mixture might still be crumbly and that is okay.

4. Press the curst into the baking dish and bake for about 15 minutes.

5. Meanwhile, prepare the filling by combining all the listed ingredients and use the electric mixer to make it easier to get a smooth consistency.

6. When you remove the crust from the oven, pour the lemon mixture on it and place back in the oven for another 15 minutes or so.

7. When done, let it cool down completely before cutting and serving.

Nutrition Information per serving: 90 Calories, 6 g total fat, 57 mg cholesterol, 52 mg sodium, **3 g carbonates (sugars),** 0.8g fiber, and 3.1g protein.

YOU NEW FAVORITE CHOCOLATE COOKIES

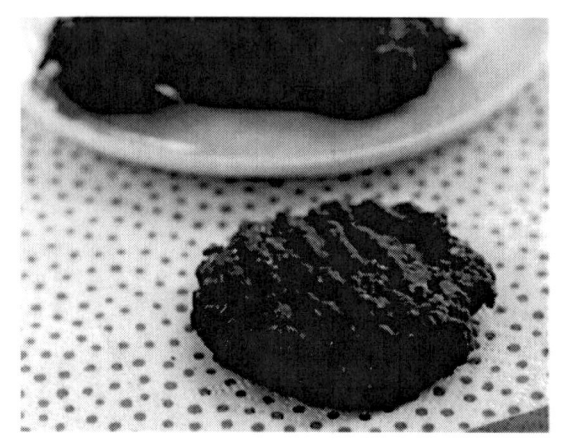

Makes:
24 Servings

Preparation time:
45 minutes

Ingredients:
½ cup unsweetened cocoa powder
Pinch of salt
½ cup stevia (divided)
1 tsp. pure almond extract
1 Tbsp. almond flour
1 Tbsp. coconut palm sugar
1/8 tsp. cream of tartar
3 medium eggs

Directions:

1. Preheat the oven to 325 degrees F.
2. In a bowl, combine the cocoa powder, ¼ cup Stevia and salt.
3. In a different mixing bowl, use the electric mixer once again to beat the eggs and the cream of tartar, as well as the rest of the stevia.
4. Finally, add the first chocolate mixture and stir again.
5. Use a teaspoon to drop the chocolate dough on a greased baking sheet.
6. Bake in the oven for about 30 minutes.

Nutrition Information per serving: 25 Calories, 0.9 g total fat, 3 mg cholesterol, 13 mg sodium, **6 g carbonates (sugars),** 1g fiber, and 1.2g protein.

DARKER ANGEL FOOD CAKE

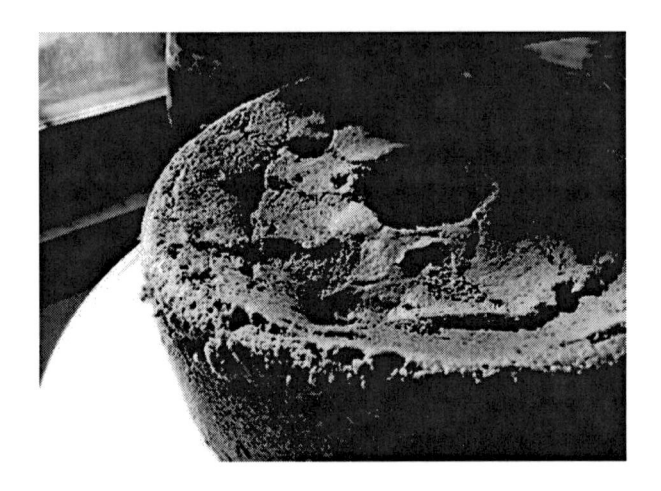

Makes:
10-12 Servings

Preparation time:
1.5 hour

Ingredients:
1 cup almond flour
½ cup quinoa flour
1 cup powered sweet proteins such as Monelin, Curculin
⅓ cup unsweetened cocoa powder
½ tsp. ground nutmeg
9 eggs whites (room temperature)
1 tsp. cream of tartar
1Tbsp. pure almond extract

Directions:
1. Preheat the oven to 375 degrees F.

2. In a large bowl mix the dry ingredients such as flours, ½ of the suggested amount of sweet proteins sugar, cocoa powder and nutmeg.

3. With a good whisk or an electric mixer, bring the egg whites to foam. Add the cream of tartar to it, as well as the rest of the sugars and almond extract. You should continue mixing until the mixture forms some peeks.

4. Add the dry ingredients to the eggs mixture and mix well. Pour the mixture than in a greased baking cake dish of your choice. Of course, I have a weakness for the angel cake food pan.

5. Bake for about 50 minutes, double-check with a knife to make sure it comes back out clean, and then you know it's done.

Nutrition Information per serving: 125 Calories, 1 g total fat, 15 mg cholesterol, 47 mg sodium, **26 g carbonates (sugars),** 1g fiber, and 5g protein.

PEACH AND STRAWBERRIES SHAKE

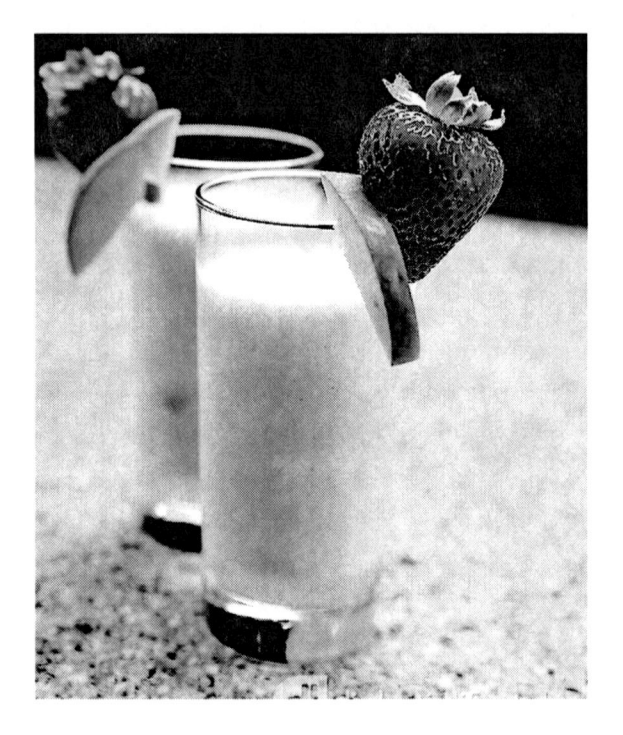

Makes:
2 Servings

Preparation time:
5 minutes

Ingredients:
2 fresh peaches (peeled, pitted and sliced)
½ cup fresh strawberries (sliced)
2 cups skim milk
Pinch ground ginger

Directions:

1. In your high speed blender place the washed and sliced peaches and strawberries.

2. Add the milk and the ginger. Activate the blender until texture is smooth enough to your taste.

3. Serve in 2 tall glasses, or save one in the fridge for later that day.

Nutrition Information per serving: 101 Calories, 0.1 g total fat, 15 mg cholesterol, 65 mg sodium, **22 g carbonates (sugars),** 3g fiber, and 5g protein.

CHOCOLATE AND COFFEE MERINGUES

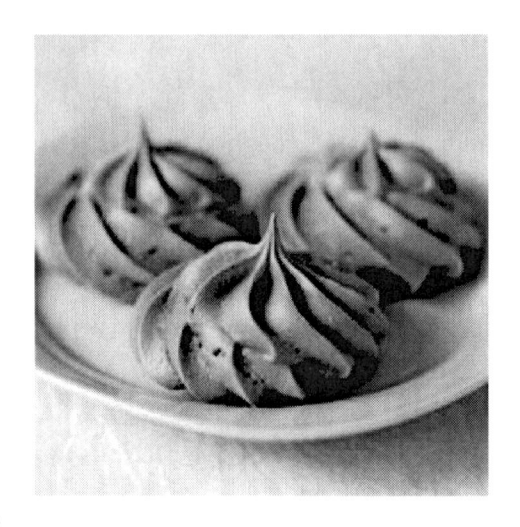

Makes:
36 Servings

Preparation time:
1 hour 20 minutes

Ingredients:
2 Tbsp. unsweetened cocoa powder
1 Tbsp. almond flour
½ tsp. instant coffee powder
3 medium egg whites
½ cup pure Stevia

Directions:
1. Preheat the oven to only 250 degrees F.

2. In a bowl, mix the cocoa powder, almond flour and coffee powder.

3. Whisk the egg whites with the sugar (add gradually) until it gets foamy, I suggest you use the electric mixer, it will be much easier.

4. Add the cocoa mixture to this last mix.

5. Drop a spoonful of mixture on the greased baking sheet and bake the meringues for about an hour.

6. You will need to let them cool off when done and get crunchy.

Nutrition Information per serving: 12 Calories, 0 g total fat, 0 mg cholesterol, 11 mg sodium, **3.2 g carbonates (sugars),** 0g fiber, and 0g protein.

BREAKFAST OR DESSERT SMOOTHIE

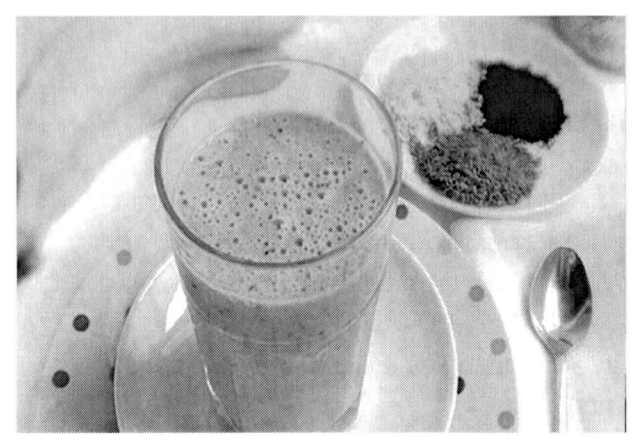

Makes:
2 Servings

Preparation time:
10 minutes

Ingredients:
2 Tbsp. coconut flour
2 Tbsp. flax seeds
2 frozen bananas
3 cups unsweetened coconut milk
1 Tbsp. sugarcane juice
Pinch ground cinnamon

Directions:
1. Of course you can always modify slightly the ingredients. If you are not a big fan of coconut milk for example, use almond or cashew milk, just make sure you use the unsweetened kind.

2. Place all the ingredients listed above in the blender.

3. Activate the blender on high speed until the mixture completely smooth and drinkable through a straw.

4. Pour in your favorite cups or glasses.

5. Cheers!

Nutrition Information per serving: 179 Calories, 1 g total fat, 101 mg cholesterol, 39 mg sodium, **17 g carbonates (sugars),** 3.1g fiber, and 1g protein.

GREEN BUT SWEET SMOOTHIE IDEA

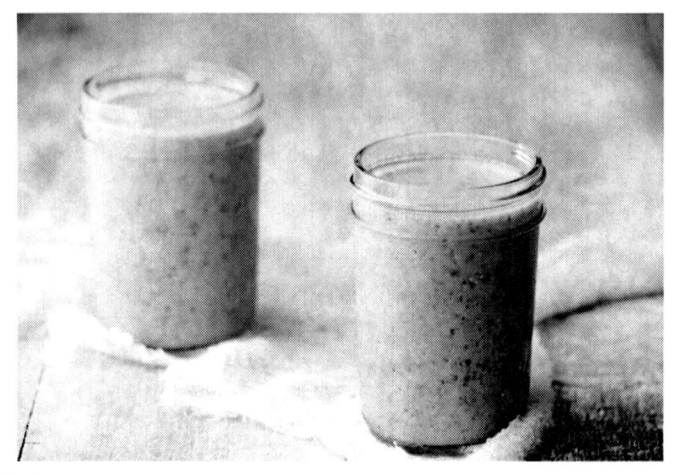

Makes:
2 Servings

Preparation time:
12 minutes

Ingredients:
2 cups unsweetened cashew milk
1 cup chopped fresh spinach
1 Tbsp. flaxseeds
¼ cup ice cubes
2 Tbsp. Manuka honey

Directions:
1. Add all the ingredients should be placed in the blender and blend until it is smooth.

2. This drink is low in carbs, but certainly loaded in antioxidants, drink up!

Nutrition Information per serving: 115 Calories, 1.3 g total fat, 15 mg cholesterol, 150 mg sodium, **24 g carbonates (sugars),** 2g fiber, and 3g protein.

CHEESE AND PEARS DELICIOUS COMBO

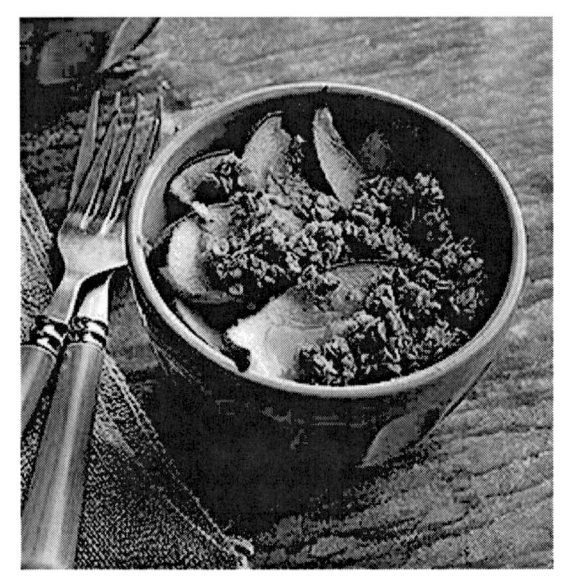

Makes:
4 Servings

Preparation time:
1.5 hour

Ingredients:
2 ripe and sliced pears, (cored also)
1 Tbsp. fresh lemon juice
1/4 cup low fat shredded sharp Cheddar cheese
½ cup coconut flour
1 Tbsp. pure Stevia
½ tsp. ground cinnamon
2 Tbsp. coconut moil (melted)

Directions:
1. Preheat oven to 425 degrees F.

2. Simply place the sliced pears on the bottom of a greased baking dish and drizzle the lemon juice on them.

3. Sprinkle the shredded cheese on top of the pears.

4. In a small bowl, prepare the crust by mixing the coconut flour, Stevia, cinnamon and coconut oil.

5. Finally sprinkle the coconut flour's mixture on top of the dish and bake in the oven for about 20 minutes.

6. Remove from the oven when the cheese is completely melted.

Nutrition Information per serving: 202 Calories, 5 g total fat, 25 mg cholesterol, 160 mg sodium, **23 g carbonates (sugars),** 3.9g fiber, and 7g protein.

ZUCCHINI CHOCOLATE BREAD

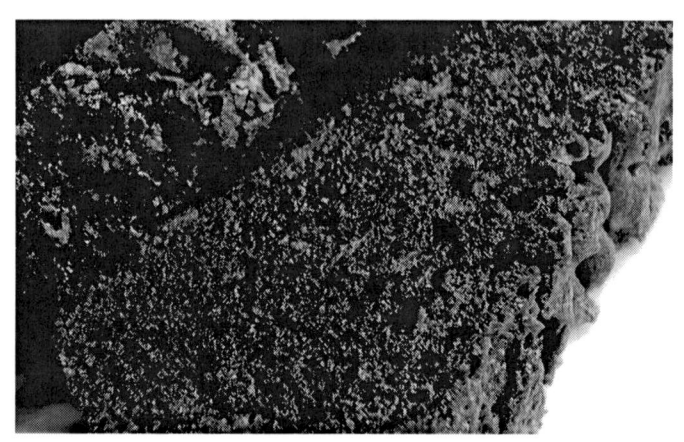

Makes:
16 Servings

Preparation time:
1.5 hour

Ingredients:
1 cup shredded zucchinis (1 medium)
⅔ Cup Manuka honey
⅔ cup unsweetened cocoa powder
½ cup apple juice
2 medium eggs
2 cup almond flour
1 tsp.; baking powder
1 tsp. baking soda
1 tsp. ginger
1 tsp. all spices
Pinch salt

Directions:
1. Preheat the oven to 350 degrees F.

2. In a mixing bowl, combine the dry ingredients including the almond flour, baking powder and soda, the salt, ginger, all spices.

3. In a medium saucepan, place the apple juice, the cocoa power and honey. Heat on low until all is mixed well and set aside.

4. Add the eggs into the chocolate cooled down mixture.

5. Incorporate next the almond flour mixture into the chocolate one and stir until no lumps are seen.

6. Finally, add the shredded zucchinis and mix again.

7. Pour the chocolate batter into a greased cake or bread pan, depending on your mood.

8. Bake for about 55 minutes to an hour.

9. Let it cool down before slicing and tasting.

Nutrition Information per serving: 115 Calories, 1.3 g total fat, 15 mg cholesterol, 150 mg sodium, **24 g carbonates (sugars),** 2g fiber, and 3g protein.

BANANA FRENCH TOASTS EGGS FREE

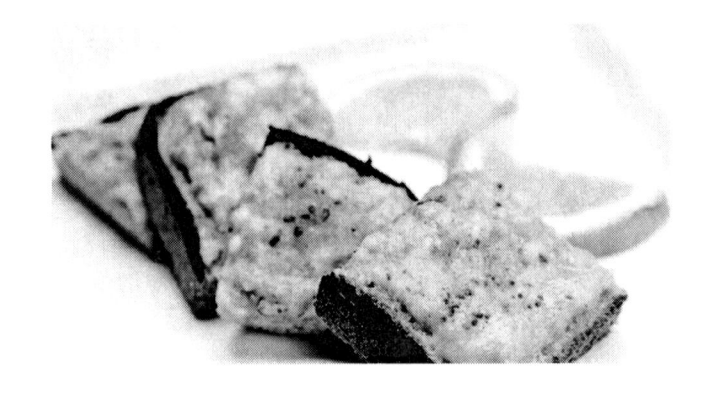

Makes:
2 Servings

Preparation time:
15 minutes

Ingredients:
1 ripe banana
1 tablespoon fresh lime or lemon juice
¼ teaspoon ground nutmeg
2 slices of diabetic friendly bread (light Tapioca or almond flour bread)
Coconut oil

Directions:
1. In a small bowl, whisk the ripe banana and the lemon juice with nutmeg.

2. You are basically making the equivalent of French toasts but with no eggs.

3. Heat coconut oil on medium heat in a skillet.

4. Dip the slices of brad in your banana mix.

5. Cook the bread on each side until golden.

6. You can cut the bread in quarters for finger bites.

Nutrition Information per serving: 132 Calories, 2 g total fat, 0 mg cholesterol, 149 mg sodium, **27 g carbonates (sugars),** 4g fiber, and 4g protein.

CHOCOLATE AND CHERRIES LOW CARBS CAKE

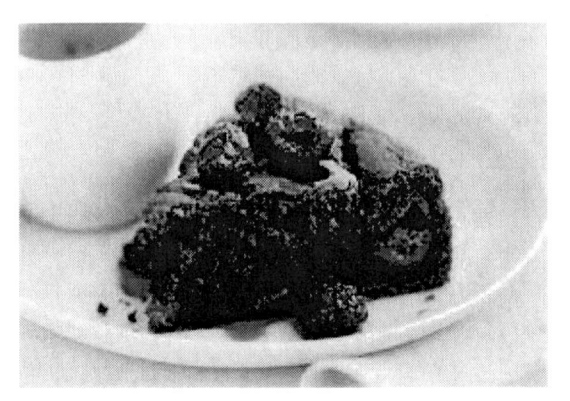

Makes:
10- 12 Servings

Preparation time:
1.5 hour

Ingredients:
2 cups quinoa flour
1 cup pure Stevia
½ cup unsweetened cocoa powder
2 Tbsp. coconut oil
2 large eggs
1 tsp. pure vanilla
1 tsp. baking powder
½ tsp. baking soda
Pinch salt
1 1/2 cup fresh cherries (pitted)
½ cup sugar free cherry jam

Some water

Directions:
1. Always preheat the oven first to 350 degrees F.

2. Mix the following together: flour, Stevia, cocoa powder, salt, baking soda, baking powder in a large mixing bowl.

3. In another bowl, combine the yoghurt, the coconut oil, and vanilla.

4. Whish the eggs and add them to the yoghurt mixture, stir well.

5. Finally, gradually incorporate the wet mixture into the dry one until the batter is ready and lumps free.

6. Pour the batter into a square greased baking dish and bake for about 40 minutes.

7. Meanwhile in small saucepan, heat up the cherries, cherries jam and water. Mix together well.

8. Once the cake is done, let it cool down.

9. When serving, pour some of the cherries mixture on top.

Nutrition Information per serving: 201 Calories, 3.3 g total fat, 111 mg cholesterol, 178 mg sodium, **40 g carbonates (sugars),** 3g fiber, and 5g protein.

THE PERFECT LOW SUGARS FLAN

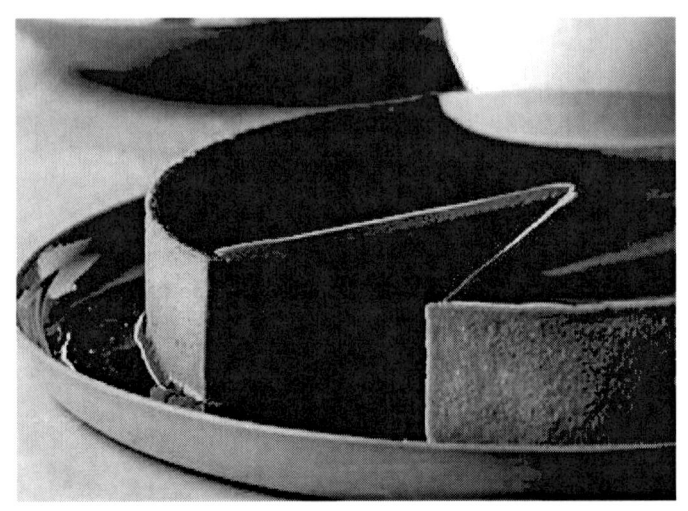

Makes:
6 Servings

Preparation time:
2 hours

Ingredients:
4 cups skim milk
¼ c unsweetened cocoa powder
1/2 tsp. ground cinnamon
½ tsp. nutmeg
1 cup coconut palm sugar
1 tsp. almond extract
4 large eggs
3 Tbsp. tab water

Directions:

1. Preheat the oven to 350 degrees F please.

2. In a large pot, combine the skim milk, cocoa powder, cinnamon, nutmeg and ½ cup coconut palm sugar, while setting the temperature on medium heat.

3. Continue cooking for about 20 minutes, and stir frequently. Set aside.

4. In a different saucepan, also mix the remaining of coconut palm sugar and water. Bring to boil so it dissolves completely and gets thicker. You will want to cook the syrup until it darkens, it will be your top coat.

5. Grease either a large round baking dish or 4 small dishes you can place in a large dish, oven safe.

6. Final step is to whisk the eggs and add the milk mixture gradually and the almond extract and then pour into the greased dish.

7. Add the syrup you created on top and bake for about 40 minutes or so. The flan should be firm when you get it out of the oven.

8. Let it cool down before serving or cutting.

Nutrition Information per serving: 250 Calories, 5.3 g total fat, 150 mg cholesterol, 119 mg sodium, **34 g carbonates (sugars),** 1g fiber, and 10g protein.

NO FLOUR VANILLA AND ALMOND CAKE

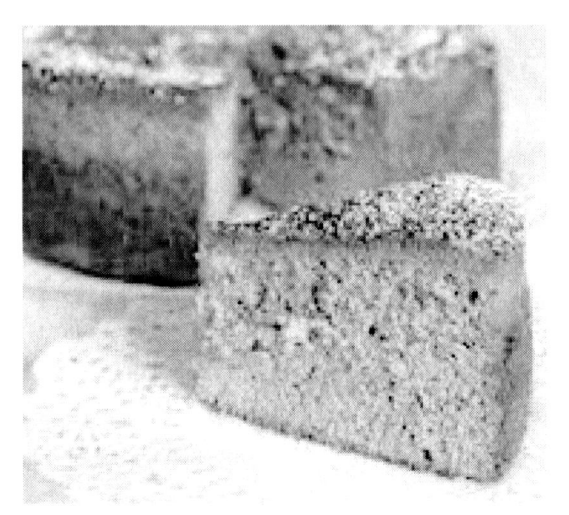

Makes:
10-12 Servings

Preparation time:
1 hour

Ingredients:
3 Tbsp. unsweetened vanilla proteins powder
1 cup raw sliced almonds
1 cup coconut palm sugar (divided)
½ cup low fat sour cream
1 Tbsp. coconut oil
2 large egg yolks
1 Tbsp. almond extract
5 large egg whites (room temperature)
Pinch salt

Directions:
1. Preheat the oven to 350 degrees F. Also prepare a cake baking pan with either coconut oil or cooking spray.

2. In the food processor, grind the almonds until it becomes powdery.

3. Mix the proteins powder with a little water and then add the grinded almonds, the sour cream, the egg yolks, coconut oil, ½ cup coconut palm sugar and almond extract, in large amount.

4. Next step is to combine the egg whites and salt and using an electric mixer, to mix until peaks form.

5. Transfer the eggs whites into the proteins powder mixture and fold.

6. Pour the new mixture into the can pan and bake for about 35 minutes.

7. Once done, let the cake cool down. You can also sprinkle some coconut palm sugar on top.

Nutrition Information per serving: 175 Calories, 3.3 g total fat, 20 mg cholesterol, 84 mg sodium, **21 g carbonates (sugars),** 2g fiber, and 4g protein.

CHOCOLATE COOKIES WITH PEPPERMINT SPLASH

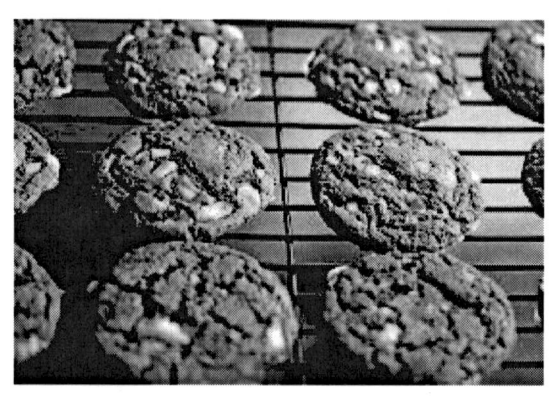

Makes:
36 Servings

Preparation time:
1 hour

Ingredients:
1/2 cup grass fed butter (room temperature)
3/4 cup pure stevia
1 large egg
1 tsp. almond extract
1/3 cup unsweetened cocoa
2 cups quinoa flour
1 tsp. Baking powder
1 tsp. baking soda
Pinch salt
½ crushed peppermint candies (sugar free kind)

Directions:
1. Preheat oven to 350 degrees F.

2. With an electric mixer, mix the butter, adding the sugar and mix until it's creamy.

3. Add the egg and almond extract next. Mix well.

4. Add also the quinoa flour, the baking soda, baking powder, salt to the original mixture.

5. Finally add the crushed peppermint candy in your batter.

6. Drop one tablespoon at a time or if you want to make them smaller, a teaspoon at a time on a previously greased cookie sheet.

7. Bake in the oven for about 12 minutes.

8. Cool down and bite into this Holiday like cookie.

Nutrition Information per serving: 75 Calories, 2.7 g total fat, 20 mg cholesterol, 90 mg sodium, **12 g carbonates (sugars),** 0.2g fiber, and 1.2g protein.

A SIMPLY DELICIOUS PINEAPPLE CAKE

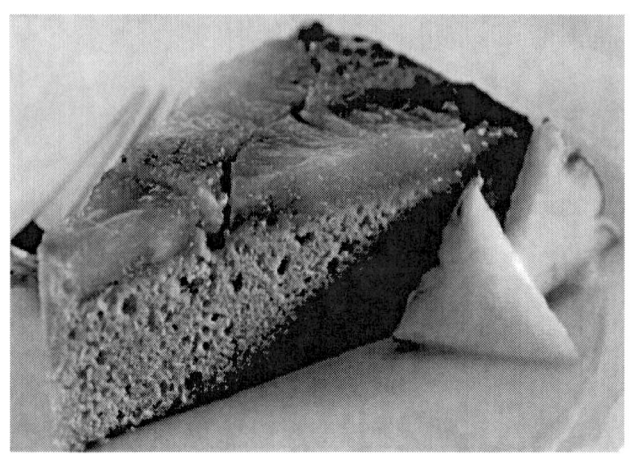

Makes:
12 Servings

Preparation time:
1 hour

Ingredients:
1 can unsweetened pineapple slices (keep the juice also)
2 Tbsp. Manuka honey
1 tsp. cinnamon
1 cup coconut palm sugar
¼ cup coconut oil (room temperature)
2 egg whites
1/2 teaspoon pure vanilla
1 ½ cup almond flour
1/2 teaspoon baking soda

Directions:
1. Preheat oven to 375 degrees F.

2. Choose the cake pan you like and grease it with some coconut oil. Set aside.

3. Separate the pineapple slices from its juice. Place the pineapple slices in the very bottom of the pan. You guessed it; it will be an upside down cake.

4. Drizzle the honey on the fruits and also sprinkle evenly the cinnamon. Set aside.

5. In a large mixing bowl, combine the egg whites, vanilla, coconut palm sugar and coconut oil. Add the dry ingredients next: almond flour, baking soda and also the pineapple juice. Mix well. Take out your electric mixer if you like to do so.

6. Once well mixed, pour the batter on top of the pineapple slices and bake in the oven for about 30 minutes.

7. You will enjoy this delicious fruity cake.

Nutrition Information per serving: 165 Calories, 4 g total fat, 0 mg cholesterol, 108 mg sodium, **27 g carbonates (sugars),** 2g fiber, and 1g protein.

A CHOCOLATE BREAD DELIGHT IDEA

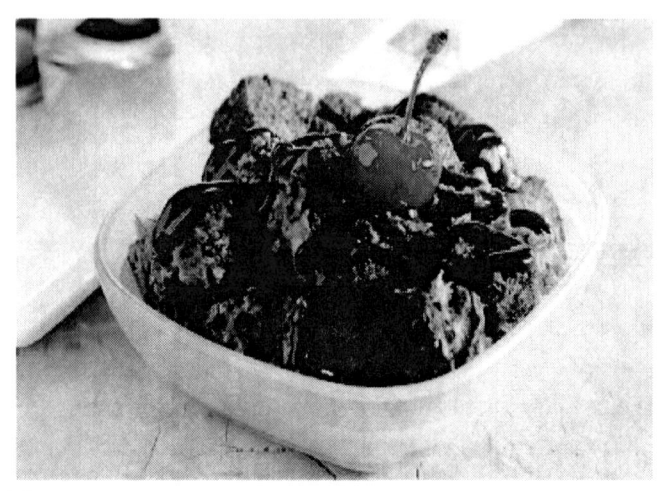

Makes:
8 Servings

Preparation time:
1 hour

Ingredients:
1/4 cup pure Stevia
2 Tbsp. unsweetened cocoa powder
1 1/2 cups unsweetened almond milk
3 large
1 tsp. lemon zest
1 tsp. pure almond extract
1 tsp. ground cinnamon
4 cubes whole grains bread or sourdough bread
Optional: store bought 1 chocolate syrup

Directions:

1. Preheat oven to 350 degrees F.

2. In a large bowl, combine the stevia, cocoa. Add the almond milk, eggs, almond extract, cinnamon and lemon zest.

3. In a greased large baking pan (coconut oil works), place all the bread cubes.

4. Add the milk mixture and bake for about 40 minutes.

5. Serve warm and drizzle some sugar free chocolate syrup if you choose to.

Nutrition Information per serving: 130 Calories, 2 g total fat, 130 mg cholesterol, 80 mg sodium, **23 g carbonates (sugars),** 1g fiber, and 6g protein.

CRANBERRY PINEAPPLE BREAD PUDDING

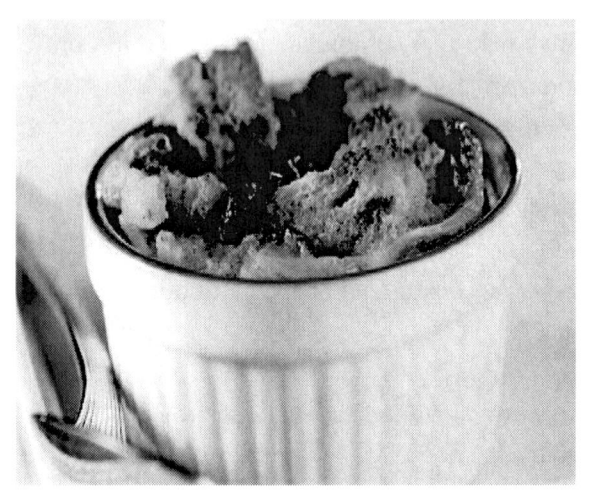

Makes:
9 Servings

Preparation time:
50 minutes

Ingredients:
2 cups cinnamon swirl or sugar free chocolate swirl bread (cubes)
1/4 cup dried cranberries
2 cups unsweetened coconut milk
2 scoops sugar free vanilla proteins powder
2 eggs
1 can pineapples sugar free (cubes)
1 tsp. ground cinnamon

Directions:
1. Preheat oven to 350 degrees F.

2. You can choose to prepare this dish in individual oven safe cups or a large dish. Let's choose a large baking pan for this example.

3. Grease the rectangle baking dish with coconut oil and place the bread cubes evenly on the bottom of it.

4. On top of the bread also pour the pineapple cubes and cranberries.

5. In a large mixing bowl, combine the rest of the ingredients and stir. Then, pour the custard created on top.

6. Bake for 35 minutes and serve warm with fresh cream if you like.

Nutrition Information per serving: 75 Calories, 1 g total fat, 2 mg cholesterol, 180 mg sodium, **11 g carbonates (sugars),** 1g fiber, and 4g protein.

THE PERFECT CAKE DUO: CHOCOLATE AND PUMPKIN

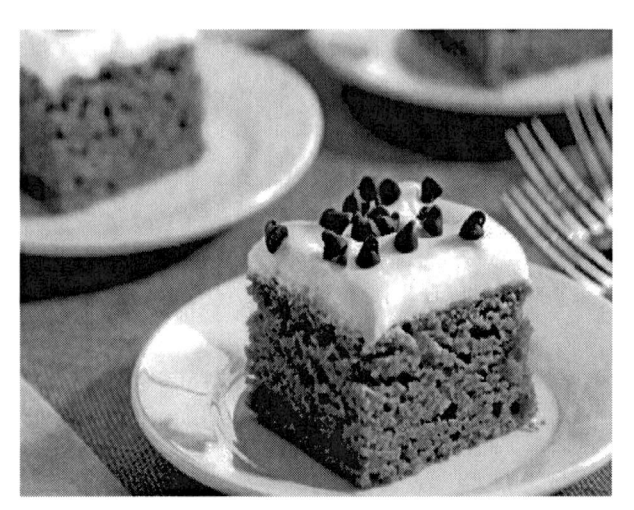

Makes:

24 Servings

Preparation time:

1 hour

Ingredients:

1 cup tapioca flour

1 cup coconut flour

3/4 cup coconut palm sugar

1 tsp. baking powder

1 tsp. baking soda

2 tsp. all spices

1 can sugar free pumpkin puree

3 medium eggs

¼ coconut oil (room temperature)

3 Tbsp. sugarcane syrup
1 ½ cup fat free cream cheese (room temperature)
2 additional Tbsp. coconut palm sugar
¼ cup unsweetened chocolate chips

Directions:
1. Preheat oven to 325 degrees F.

2. Use a mixing bowl to combine the dry ingredients: flours, coconut pal sugar, baking soda, baking powder and spices.

3. In a different bowl, mix the wet ingredients: pumpkin puree, eggs, coconut oil, and sugarcane syrup.

4. Combine both mixtures and stir until the texture is super smooth.

5. Pour the batter in a large square dish and bake for about 30 minutes.

6. Time to make the cheese frosting: in a bowl, use the electric mixer to bring to a fluffy texture the cream cheese and 2 tbsp. Coconut palm sugar.

7. When the cake is cooked, frost it with the cream cheese frosting and sprinkle of chocolate chips.

Nutrition Information per serving: 170 Calories, 4 g total fat, 20 mg cholesterol, 170 mg sodium, **15 g carbonates (sugars),** 2g fiber, and 3g protein.

MANGO CREPES

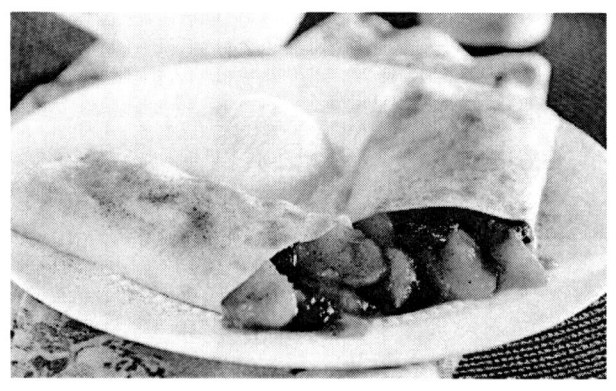

Makes:
4 Servings

Preparation time:
1 hour

Ingredients:
1 ripe mango (peeled, pitted, cubed)
¼ cup dried golden raisins
2 tsp. lemon juice
½ tsp. nutmeg
½ tsp. cinnamon
2 Tbsp. walnut oil
1/4 cup low sugar mango or orange juice
1 Tbsp. pure stevia
3/4 teaspoon cornstarch
½ tsp. vanilla extract
4 prepared already crêpes (almond or coconut flour)

Directions:

1. In a large saucepan, cook on medium/low heat the mango, walnut oil, dried raisins with lemon juice and spices for about 30 minutes.

2. Meanwhile, you should prepare your favorite crepes recipe. (Keep warm in the oven)

3. Also, in a small saucepan, you will prepare the syrup for the mango crepes: mix the mango juice with the stevia, cornstarch and vanilla.

4. Start setting up the crepes. One per person, with generous filling of mango mixture. Fold it and drizzle a tablespoon of the syrup on top.

5. Enjoy for dessert or a very delicious breakfast.

Nutrition Information per serving: 240 Calories, 9 g total fat, 100 mg cholesterol, 221 mg sodium, **32 g carbonates (sugars),** 3g fiber, and 6g protein.

SUGARCANE FLAVORED CUSTARD

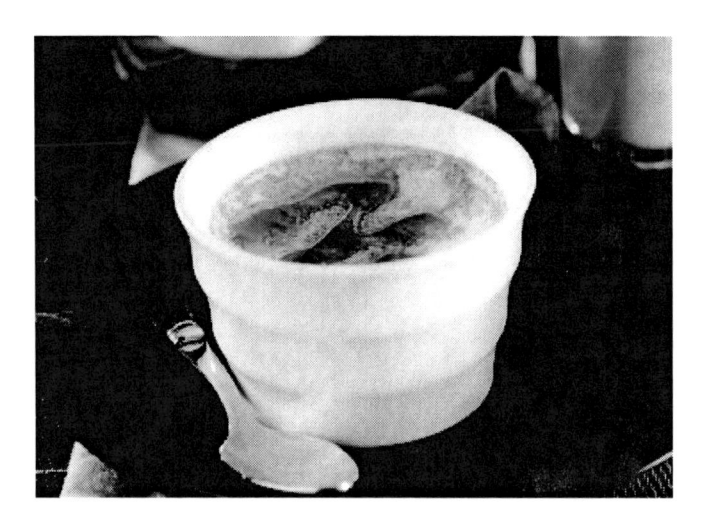

Makes:
6 Servings

Preparation time:
1 hour

Ingredients:
2 cups heavy cream
2 eggs
¼ cup coconut palm sugar
2 Tbsp. sugarcane syrup
3 cups boiling water
Pinch cinnamon

Directions:
1. Preheat oven to 300 degrees F.

2. Prepare 6 small oven-safe ramequins with non-stick cooking spray.

3. In a bowl, mix the heavy cream, eggs, coconut palm sugar, and cinnamon.

4. Pour the mixture equally into each ramequin.

5. Pour the boiling water into a large rectangle dish and place the ramequins inside.

6. Bake for a little over an hour.

7. Combine half-and-half, egg substitute, sugar, vanilla, and nutmeg in large bowl. Pour into prepared custard cups.

8. Serve with some sugarcane syrup on top, if you wish.

Nutrition Information per serving: 130 Calories, 1 g total fat, 20 mg cholesterol, 139 mg sodium, **23 g carbonates (sugars),** 0g fiber, and 5.1g protein.

CHOCOLATE CREPES WITH FRUITS

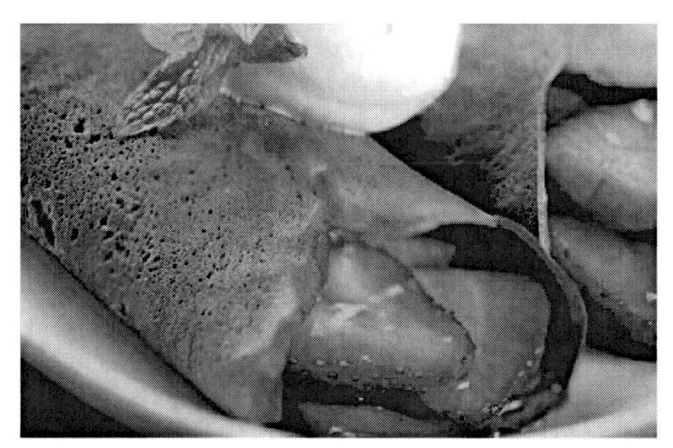

Makes:
8 Servings

Preparation time:
1 hour

Ingredients:
1 cup quinoa flour
1 cup cashew milk
2 Tbsp. unsweetened cocoa powder
3 egg whites
2 Tbsp. pure Stevia
2 Tbsp. coconut oil
3 cups of your favorite berries: blueberries, strawberries, raspberries, blackberries...
2 Tbsp. Manuka honey
Pinch salt

Directions:
1. Let's prepare the chocolate crepes first.

2. Combine the quinoa flour, eggs whites, Stevia, coconut oil and cocoa powder. Stir for a while until the mixture is smooth.

3. Heat coconut oil in a small skillet and pour enough for a crepe at a time. Cook as many crepes as you will need.

4. Meanwhile, in a small saucepan, place the berries chosen with a few tablespoons of water and 2 Tbsp. of Manuka honey. Bring to a boil and then set aside.

5. Start filing each chocolate crepe when ready with the berries mixture. Serve warm.

Nutrition Information per serving: 280 Calories, 8 g total fat, 56 mg cholesterol, 387 mg sodium, **52 g carbonates (sugars),** 5g fiber, and 9g protein.

DELECTABLE PEANUT COOKIES

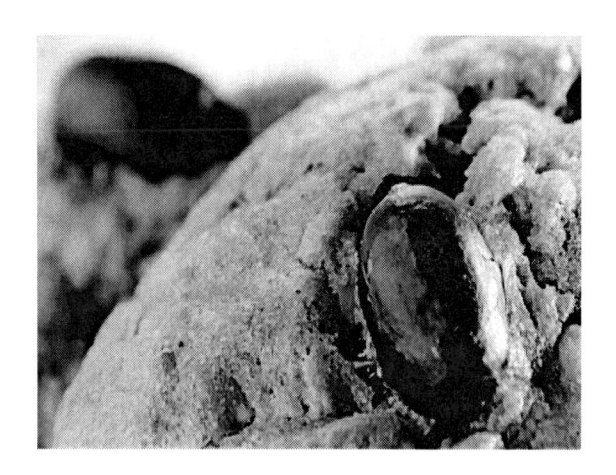

Makes:
24 Servings

Preparation time:
1 hour

Ingredients:
¼ cup coconut or walnut oil
¾ natural no sugar added peanut butter
¼ cup unsweetened apple juice
1 cup quinoa flour
1 Tbsp. flaxseeds
1 egg
1 tsp. almond extract
1 tsp. baking soda
Pinch salt
¼ cup raw peanuts (optional)

Directions:
1. Preheat oven to 350 degrees F.

2. In a large mixing bowl, mix the butter, peanut butter well. Then add the egg, apple juice, almond extract.

3. Finally add the rest of the ingredients: flour, flaxseeds, baking soda and salt. If you choose to add peanuts, it's time to add them as well.

4. Mix well and then on a greased cookie sheet, place teaspoons full of dough. You should have batter for about 24 cookies, so you might need 2 baking sheets.

5. Bake for 10 minutes. Enjoy with a glass of skim milk.

Nutrition Information per serving: 100 Calories, 3 g total fat, 10 mg cholesterol, 88 mg sodium, **9 g carbonates (sugars),** 1g fiber, and 3g protein.

SWEET TEA FOR DESSERT

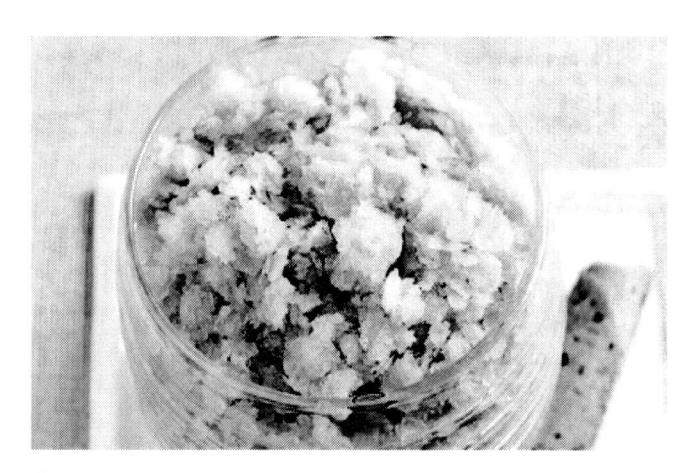

Makes:
4 Servings

Preparation time:
50 minutes

Ingredients:
Pinch ground cinnamon
Pinch ground ginger
3 cups water
4 green or black tea bags (your favorite)
2 cups unsweetened coconut milk
3 Tbsp. pure sugarcane syrup

Directions:
1. Boil the 3 cups of water in a medium pot and add the tea and the spices. Let is simmer for about 12-15 minutes.

2. Remove the tea bags and then add the coconut milk, and the sugarcane syrup.

3. Stir well and keep warm until serving, if you wish to serve it warm.

4. If you would like to transform this drink into a frozen one, cover the liquid and freeze it for about 1 hour and then use a fork to break the frozen drink into crystals.

5. Very refreshing during the summer season.

Nutrition Information per serving: 93 Calories, 0.2 g total fat, 2 mg cholesterol, 58 mg sodium, **20 g carbonates (sugars),** 0g fiber, and 4g protein.

CUPCAKES FROM THE ISLANDS

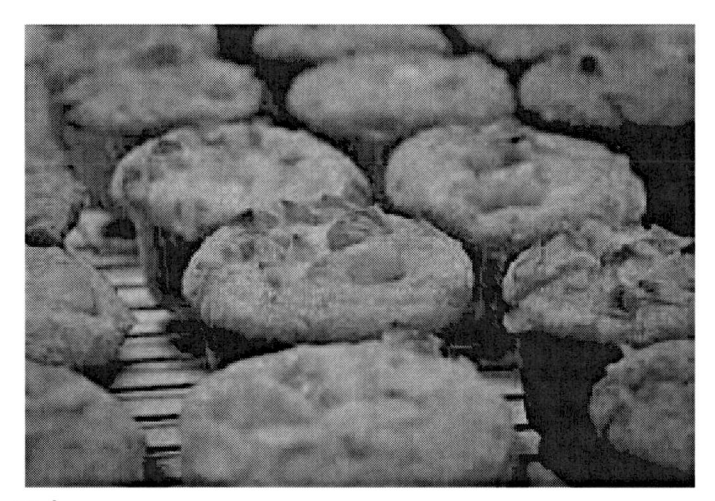

Makes:
24 Servings

Preparation time:
1 hour

Ingredients:
1 package sugar free white cake mix
1 can unsweetened crushed pineapple with their juice
2 eggs whites
1 Tbsp. coconut oil (room temperature)
½ cup shredded unsweetened coconut
1 Tbsp. orange zest
1 Tbsp. lemon juice
1 Tbsp. chia seeds

Directions:
1. Preheat oven to 350 degrees or whatever the cake mix package instructs you.

2. Greased 24 muffin tins ahead and set aside.

3. In a large bowl, combine the cake mix, egg whites, coconut oil, lemon juice and orange zest. You can use a wooden spoon or the electric mixer if you prefer.

4. Pour the batter in the muffin tins evenly. Sprinkle with chia seeds before placing in the oven

5. Bake for about 15-20 minutes.

6. Meanwhile, prepare the topping by mixing in a skillet on medium heat the crushed pineapples, the juice and shredded coconut. Cook for 10 minutes or until you are happy with the color of the coconut. It will caramelized and will make the perfect topping once your cupcakes have cooled down. Yummy!

Nutrition Information per serving: 144 Calories, 2 g total fat, 9 mg cholesterol, 155 mg sodium, **24 g carbonates (sugars),** 1g fiber, and 5g protein.

SUPER CLASSIC BREAD PUDDING

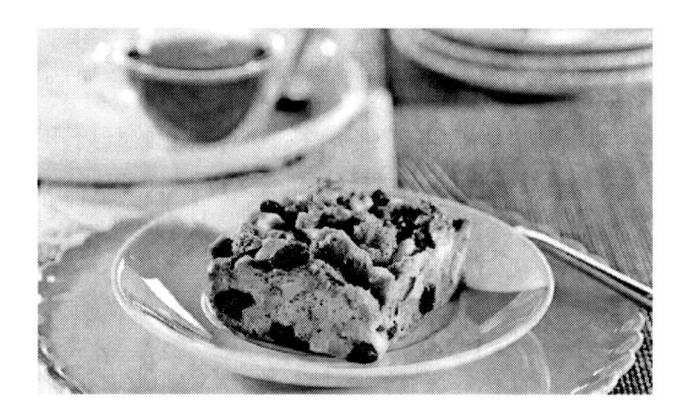

Makes:
8-12 Servings

Preparation time:
55 minutes

Ingredients:
2 cups unsweetened almond milk
4 egg whites
3 Tbsp. coconut palm sugar
2 Tbsp. melted coconut oil
1 tsp. almond extract
12 sliced of whole wheat with cinnamon swirl cut into cubes
3/4 cup dried cherries

Directions:
1. Preheat oven to 350 degrees F.

2. I like to prepare a square baking dish by greasing it with coconut oil.

3. In a large bowl, mix the egg whites, coconut palm sugar, almond extract, and almond milk.

4. When the mixture is smooth add, the bread cubes and then the dried cherries. Let it soak for about 10 minutes.

5. Pour everything into the greased dish and bake in the oven for 40 minutes.

Nutrition Information per serving: 150 Calories, 2 g total fat, 2 mg cholesterol, 214 mg sodium, **26 g carbonates (sugars),** 1g fiber, and 6g protein.

SOUR CREAM AND NUTS CAKE

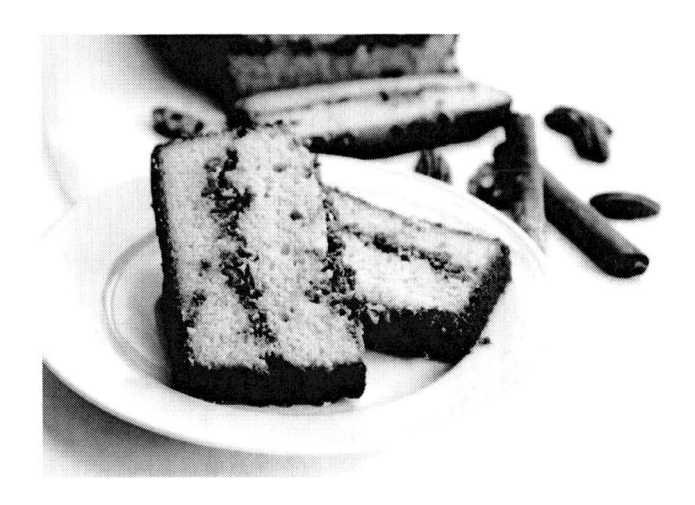

Makes:
12-16 Servings

Preparation time:
1.5 hour

Ingredients:
1/2 cup unsweetened pear & apple sauce (you can buy it in stores by applesauce)
½ cup coconut oil (room temperature)
3/4 cup pure Stevia
2 large eggs
1 cup fat-free sour cream
1 Tbsp. Manuka honey
1 1/2 cups almond flour
1 1/2 cups coconut flour
1 tsp. baking powder
½ tsp. baking soda

Pinch salt
2 Tbsp. coconut palm sugar
1 tsp. ground cinnamon
1/2 cup chopped almonds

Directions:
1. Preheat oven to 350 degrees F.

2. Mix together first the coconut oil, pear and apple sauce, sure stevia in a large bowl.

3. Add to the dry mixture the eggs, sour cream and honey. Use the electric mixer to facilitate mixing until it is smooth.

4. Next add the coconut and almond flours, baking soda, baking powder and salt.

5. Finally, prepare the middle section by mixing in a separate bowl the almonds, cinnamon and some the coconut palm sugar.

6. Pour half of the batter first into a greased square pan and then sprinkle with the nuts mixture.

7. Pour the other half of the batter and bake for about 50 minutes or until done.

Nutrition Information per serving: 180 Calories, 4 g total fat, 35 mg cholesterol, 200 mg sodium, **26 g carbonates (sugars),** 2g fiber, and 4g protein.

CHERRY DELIGHT

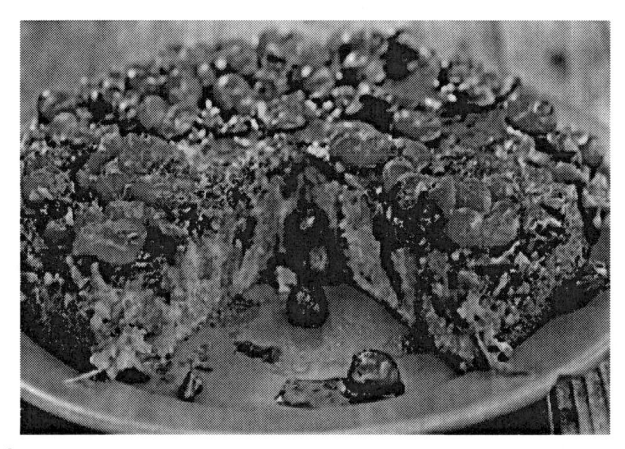

Makes:
10 Servings

Preparation time:
45 minutes

Ingredients:
2 Tbsp. non salted butter
1/2 cup fresh pitted cherries
1 cup coconut palm sugar
1/4 cup chopped walnuts
1 cup quinoa flour
1 tsp. baking powder
½ tsp. salt
1 tsp. allspices
2 large eggs
1 cup unsweetened soy milk
1 Tbsp. pure sugar cane syrup
¼ cup coconut oil (room temperature)

Directions:
1. Heat oven to 350 degrees F.

2. In a round baking pan, pour the melted butter all over.

3. In a bowl, mix the cherries, half of the coconut palm sugar and the walnuts.

4. Sprinkle the cherries mixture on the coconut oil on top of the butter evenly.

5. Finally, mix the remaining ingredients in a large bowl, creating the cake better.

6. Pour the batter on top of the cherries without mixing.

7. Bake for about 35 minutes. Let the cake cool down for 10 minutes before turning it upside down….Voila!

Nutrition Information per serving: 165 Calories, 4 g total fat, 2 mg cholesterol, 289 mg sodium, **17 g carbonates (sugars),** 4g fiber, and 4g protein.

PEANUT BUTTER BROWNIES

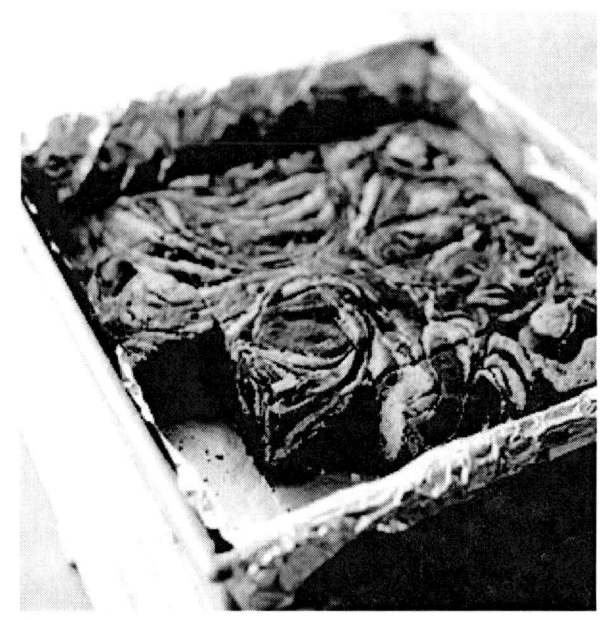

Makes:
12 Servings

Preparation time:
45 minutes

Ingredients:
¼ non-salted butter
½ cup unsweetened cocoa powder
1/3 cup sugar free peanut butter
¾ cup coconut palm sugar
¼ cup water
1/4 cup butter
2 large eggs
¼ sesame oil

1 ½ cup cashew flour (almond flour might be easier to find)
3/4 cup refrigerated or frozen egg product, thawed, or 3 eggs, lightly beaten
¼ cup unsweetened pieces of dark chocolate

Directions:
1. Preheat oven to 375 degrees F.

2. In a saucepan, combine the butter, coconut palm sugar and water on low heat. Remove from the heat and add the eggs, sesame oil and mix well.

3. Add half of the required flour in the first mixture and mix well. Set aside.

4. In a different bowl, mix the peanut butter with half of the created batter.

5. In a second bowl, do the same but with the cocoa powder.

6. You can guess you will be suing both batters to create swirls.

7. In a square greased pan, Drop by alternating peanut butter and chocolate batter and create the wanted designs.

Nutrition Information per serving: 152 Calories, 8.5 g total fat, 6 mg cholesterol, 61 mg sodium, **17.5 g carbonates (sugars),** 1g fiber, and 3.5g protein.

THE ALMOST TOO GOOD TO BE TRUE DESSERT

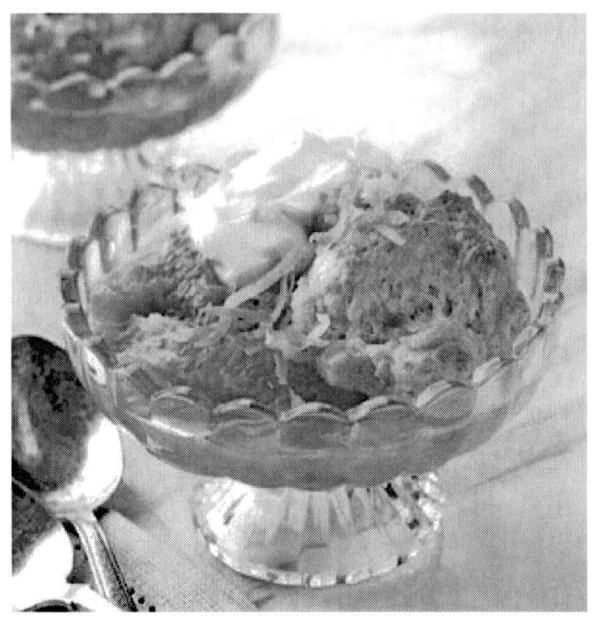

Makes:
4 Servings

Preparation time:
25 minutes

Ingredients:
4 peeled tangerines or 8 clementines (depending on the season and wat's available)
3 Tbsp. coconut palm sugar
1 tsp. ground clove
1 Tbsp. arrowroot starch
½ cup water
1 cup coconut flour
3 Tbsp. shredded coconut

Pinch nutmeg
Sugar free whipped topping (optional)

Directions:
1. Preheat oven to 425 degrees F.

2. Prepare the syrup first by mixing in a saucepan the arrowroot starch, coconut pal sugar, spices. Add gradually the water and stir until it thickens.

3. Stir in the citrus fruits (in segments of course).

4. Prepare next the topping by mixing the flour, nutmeg and the shredded coconut. Set aside.

5. Place the fruits in the bottom of a greased dish, with the topping sprinkled on top.

6. Bake for about 30 minutes. When it comes out of the oven, serve it with sugar free whipped topping

Nutrition Information per serving: 170 Calories, 3.5 g total fat, 7 mg cholesterol, 111 mg sodium, **34 g carbonates (sugars),** 3g fiber, and 4g protein.

DELICIOUS BERRIES SQUARE

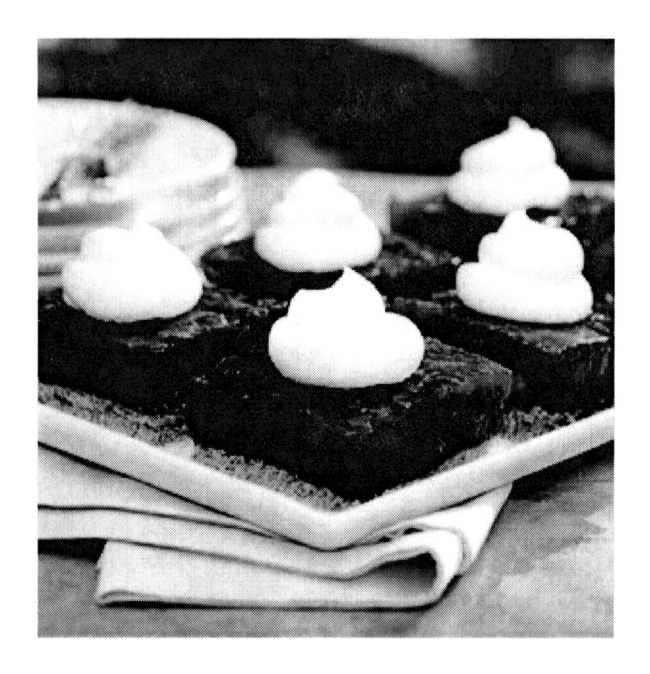

Makes:
12 Servings

Preparation time:
45 minutes

Ingredients:

Filling:

1/3 cup pure stevia

1 envelope unflavored gelatin

1 pound fresh raspberries

1 cup fresh blackberries

Crust

1 cup coconut flour
2 Tbsp. melted non salted butter
2 Tbsp. Manuka honey
Topping: sugar free whipped cream if you like

Directions:
1. Preheat oven to 400 degrees F.

2. Mix the ingredients for the crust in a bowl and then press in the bottom of a square greased baking pan. Bake for about 20 minutes. Set aside.

3. Meanwhile, let's make the filling.

4. Combine in a saucepan the berries, sugar and gelatin. Cook on medium heat and stir until all is dissolved properly. You will need to let it cool off before using it.

5. Once the crust and the filling are cooled enough, proceed by pouring the filling on top of the crust. Refrigerate for at least a few hours. When ready, cut in squares and serve with some whipped cream.

Nutrition Information per serving: 139 Calories, 4 g total fat, 7 mg cholesterol, 80 mg sodium, **25 g carbonates (sugars),** 1g fiber, and 2g protein.

HERBS AND MELON FROZEN TREATS

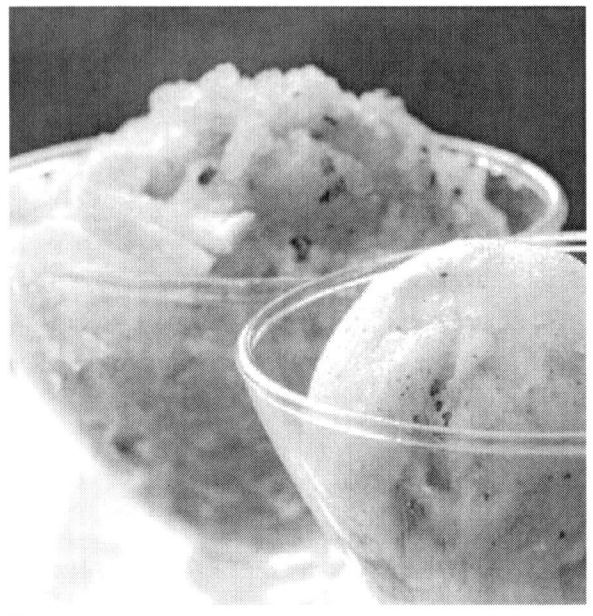

Makes:
8 Servings

Preparation time:
20 minutes + hours in freezer

Ingredients:
1/4 cup coconut palm sugar
¼ cup water
2 tbsp. Fresh chopped mint
1 Tbsp. lime juice
1 tsp. lime zest
1 medium honeydew melon (peeled, seeded and cubed)

Directions:

1. In a saucepan we will prepare the syrup first by combining the sugar and the water.

2. Bring to boil and stir until all is dissolved. Add the mint. Set aside.

3. In a high speed blender, place the melon and activate, until it is smooth.

4. Add the mint syrup you created and blend again.

5. Place the mixture in a freezer friendly container and cover with foil.

6. After about 2 or 3 hours you should be able to use a fork to scrap the mixture into crystals and serve this frozen treat in a fancy bowl or cup. Enjoy!

Nutrition Information per serving: 45 Calories, 2g total fat, 20 mg cholesterol, 10 mg sodium, **11g carbonates (sugars),** 1g fiber, and 1g protein.

STRAWBERRY AND CHEESE LOG

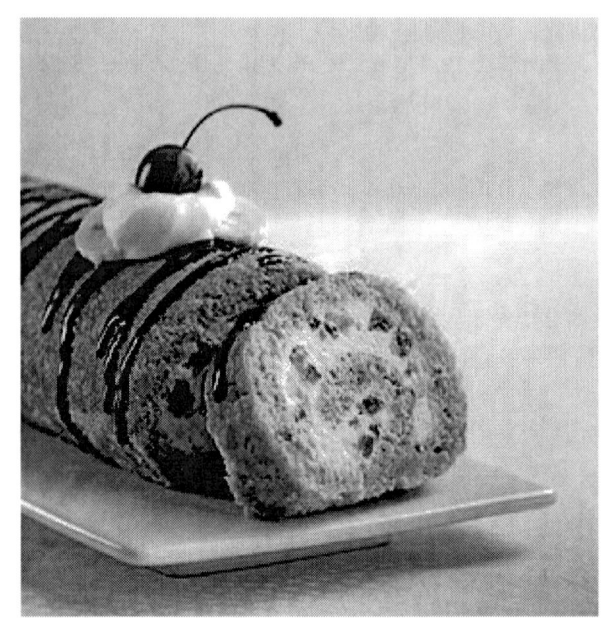

Makes:
10-12

Preparation time:
2 hours

Ingredients:
Cake
3 eggs (room temperature when ready to use)
¾ cup almond flour
1 tsp. baking powder
Pinch salt
Pinch cinnamon
¾ cup pure Stevia
1 Tbsp. orange juice

2 ripe bananas

Filling

1/3 cup sugar free whipped cream

1 package fat free cream cheese

1 cup chopped fresh strawberries

Directions:

1. Preheat your oven to 375 degrees F. Grease a rectangle baking pan with coconut oil or non-stick cooking spray. Set aside.

2. In a bowl, combine the flour, baking powder, cinnamon and salt.

3. In a different bowl, beat the eggs, I highly suggest you use an electric mixer for this one. Add gradually the Stevia, the bananas and orange juice. Finally pour the flour in the eggs mixture. Mix well and you now have your cake batter.

4. Spread the batter evenly in your greased baking pan. Bake for about 15-18 minutes.

5. When the cake comes out of the oven, remove it immediately of the dish slowly and roll it in a log by placing a towel in the middle.

6. During that time, prepare the filling by mixing all ingredients.

7. After about 45 minutes, remove the towel from the cake and unroll. Spread evenly the strawberries filling and roll the cake again.

8. Cut the cake into slices and enjoy that beautiful and delicious log cake, filled with goodness.

Nutrition Information per serving: 168 Calories, 3.5 g total fat, 69 mg cholesterol, 164 mg sodium, **28 g carbonates (sugars),** 1g fiber, and 4g protein.

SIMPLE BANANA BREAD

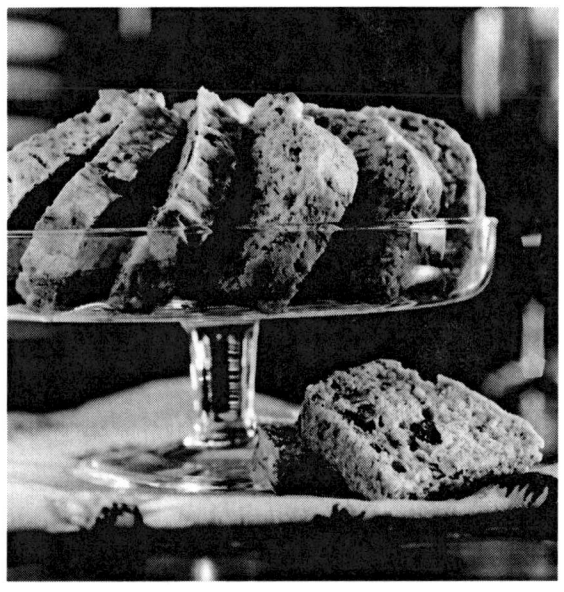

Makes:
8-10 Servings

Preparation time:
1 hour

Directions:
1 1/3 cups quinoa flour
½ cup pure Stevia
1 tsp. tsp. baking powder
½ baking soda
Pinch salt
1 Tbsp. walnut oil
1/3 cup coconut cream
2 or 3 ripe bananas

1 tsp. almond extract

1/3 cup chopped pecans

Directions:
1. Preheat oven to 350 degrees F.

2. Combine all the dry ingredients: quinoa flour, baking soda, baking powder, salt, and Stevia.

3. Next add the walnut oil, coconut cream and the bananas (mashed).

4. Add the pecans, stir some more. Then pour the batter into a loaf pan to bake.

5. Bake for about 50 minutes or until done.

Nutrition Information per serving: 160 Calories, 4.5 g total fat, 0 mg cholesterol, 170 mg sodium, **89.5 g carbonates (sugars),** 2g fiber, and 4g protein.

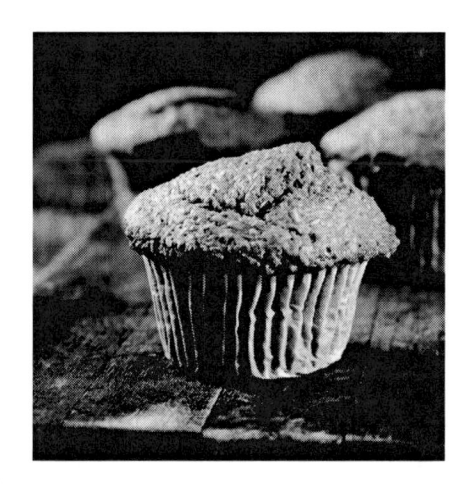

EVERYDAY MUFFINS

Makes:
12 Servings

Preparation time:
45 minutes

Ingredients:
1/4 cup unsweetened applesauce
1 large egg
2 cups unsweetened coconut milk
2 Tbsp. vanilla sugar free proteins powder.
3 tablespoons coconut oil (room temperature)
Pinch salt
3/4 cup coconut palm sugar
1 ½ cup coconut flour
½ cup flaxseeds
1 Tbsp. baking soda
1 tsp. cinnamon
Optional: Dried fruits (raisins, cranberries or cherries if you want)

Directions:
1. Preheat oven to 350 degrees F.

2. Prepare the muffins tins by greased them with coconut oil (12).

3. First combine together the egg, applesauce, coconut milk, proteins powder, coconut oil, salt and coconut palm sugar in a large bowl. Mix very well.

4. Add the rest of the ingredients and mix again until you obtain a muffin batter. If you choose to add dried fruits, add at the end and mix again.

5. Fill the muffin cups 2/3 and bake for about 25 minutes.

Nutrition Information per serving: 150 Calories, 7.5 g total fat, 20 mg cholesterol, 230 mg sodium, **22 g carbonates (sugars),** 3g fiber, and 5g protein.

SPICY CARROT BITES

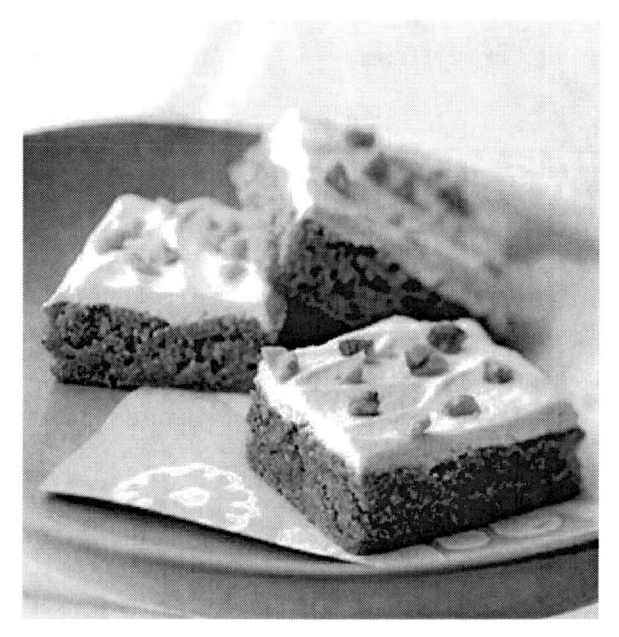

Makes:
12-16 Servings

Preparation time:
50 minutes

Ingredients:
- ¾ cup almond flour
- ½ cup pure stevia or equivalent
- 1 1/2 teaspoons pumpkin pie spice
- ½ tsp. ground ginger
- ½ tsp. ground nutmeg
- ¾ cup finely shredded carrots
- ¾ cups chopped pecans or almonds
- 2 large eggs

¼ cup unsweetened almond milk
¼ cup coconut oil (room temperature)
Frosting (optional) use sugar free of course

Directions:
1. Preheat oven to 350 degrees F.

2. First of all, in a large bowl, combine the first 5 dry ingredients. Mix well.

3. Next, add the carrots, nuts, eggs, coconut oil and almond milk. Stir well, your mixture should be ready.

4. Grease a square baking dish and pour the batter in.

5. Bake in the oven for about 20 minutes.

6. Frist with your store bought or homemade sugar free favorite frosting, if you wish.

Nutrition Information per serving: 121 Calories, 7 g total fat, 5 mg cholesterol, 61 mg sodium, **12 g carbonates (sugars),** 1g fiber, and 2.5g protein.

DRESSED UP PEACHES

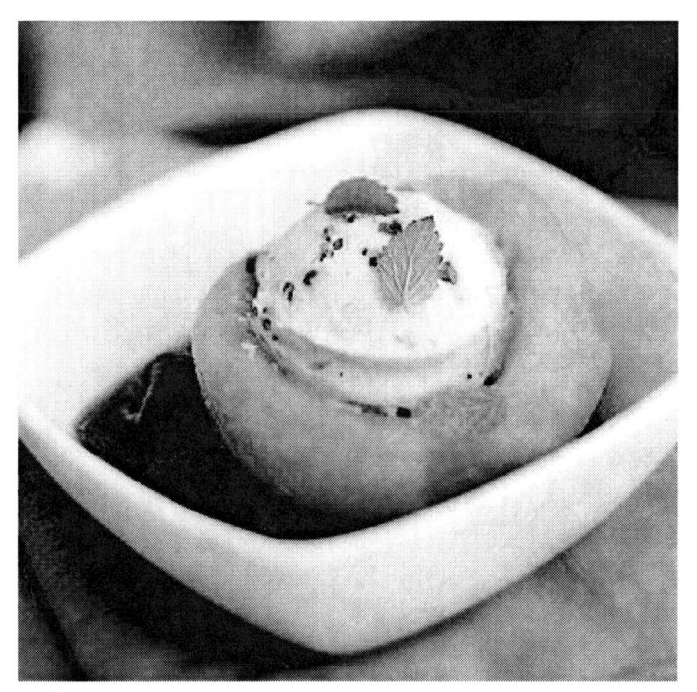

Makes:
6 Servings

Preparation time:
5 minutes

Ingredients:
¼ cup goat cheese (room temperature)
1 Tbsp. Manuka honey
Pinch nutmeg
2 Tbsp. chopped walnuts
4-6 peaches (pitted and cut in halves)

½ cup Fresh berries (blueberries, raspberries or other)
Fresh chopped mint to garnish if you like

Directions:
1. In a bowl, prepare the cheese filing by mixing the goat cheese, honey, nuts and nutmeg. Set aside in the refrigerator.

2. Place one half peach in a bowl and about one large tablespoon of fresh berries, topped by the cheese filing. Decorate with mint.

Nutrition Information per serving: 144 Calories, 6 g total fat, 0 mg cholesterol, 11 mg sodium, **21 g carbonates (sugars),** 1g fiber, and 4g protein.

CARROT MUFFINS FOR EVERYONE

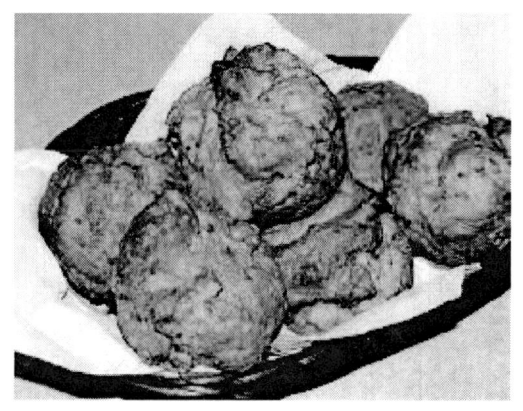

Makes:
12 Servings

Preparation time:
45 minutes

Ingredients:
1 1/3 cup quinoa flour
2 Tbsp. chai seeds
1 tsp. baking powder
1/2 tsp. baking soda
1/2 tsp. ground cinnamon
Pinch salt
1 large egg
2 large eggs
6 Tbsp. dried sweet proteins (such as Brazzein, Curculin, Mabinlin or Pentadin)
1/2 cup unsweetened pear and applesauce
1/4 cup coconut oil
2 tsp. lemon zest
1 Tbsp. sugarcane juice

1 1/2 cups shredded carrots
1/2 cup golden dried raisins

Directions:
1. Preheat oven to 350 degrees F.

2. Combine in a large bowl, the quinoa flour, chia seeds, baking powder, baking soda, salt and cinnamon.

3. In a different bowl, mix the eggs, sweet proteins. Add next the apple and pear sauce, coconut oil, lemon zest and sugarcane juice. Mix well and also add the golden raisins and carrots.

4. Finally add all dry mixture to the wet one and mix again thoroughly.

5. Fill 12 previously greased muffin cups pan almost to the top.

6. Bake for about 25-30 minutes or so.

Nutrition Information per serving: 180 Calories, 6 g total fat, 20 mg cholesterol, 10 mg sodium, 25 **g carbonates (sugars),** 2g fiber, and 3g protein.

UNIQUE RASPBERRY SOUP

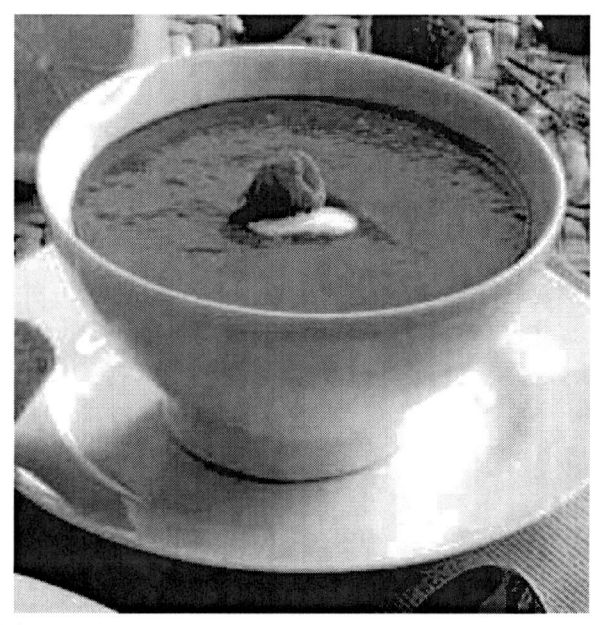

Makes:
4-6 Servings

Preparation time:
35 minutes

Ingredients:
1 ½ cup fresh raspberries
1 cup cranberry juice
¼ cup coconut palm sugar
1 Tbsp. orange juice
1 cup low fat sour cream
1/3 cup coconut cream
1 tsp. cinnamon
1 cup water

Directions:
1. In a high speed blender, mix the raspberries and the water and blend.

2. Pour the mixture into a saucepan and add also the cranberry, orange juices, as well as the coconut palm sugar and cinnamon.

3. Bring the mixture to a boil and once it boils, turn the heat down on low and let it simmer.

4. Add the coconut milk and keep it warm until it's time to serve.

5. When serving, drop a tablespoon of sour cream in each bowl, decorate with raspberries if you like.

Nutrition Information per serving: 240 Calories, 3 g total fat, 15 mg cholesterol, 50 mg sodium, **43 g carbonates (sugars),** 5g fiber, and 5g protein.

WHO WANTS SUSHI?

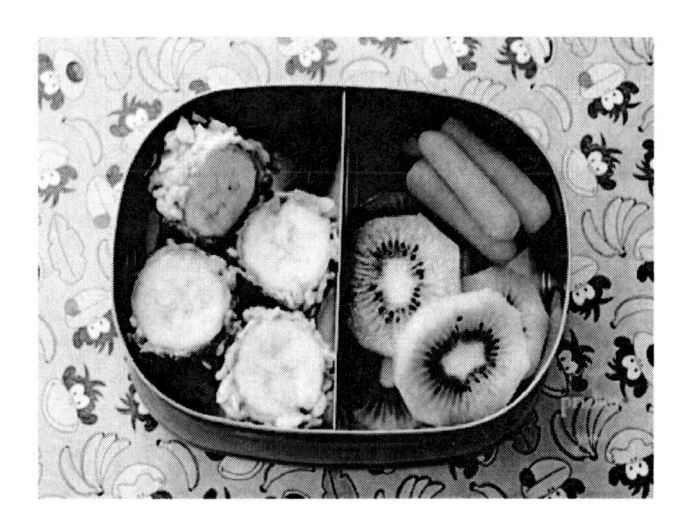

Makes:
12 Servings

Preparation time:
50 minutes

Ingredients:
2 bananas
¼ cup almond butter
1 Tbsp. coconut flour
¼ cup unsweetened coconut flakes

Directions:
1. Peel your bananas. Spread almond butter all over each banana (a nice rich coat)

2. Slice each banana in 6 thick slices.

3. Roll each "sushi piece" into the mixture of flour and coconut flakes.

4. Pack in your kid's lunch box, or serve as fun dessert bites any day of the week.

Nutrition Information per serving: 102 Calories, 1 g total fat, 12 mg cholesterol, 60 mg sodium, **15 g carbonates (sugars),** 1g fiber, and 1.2g protein.

RASPBERRIES AND POPPY SEEDS MUFFINS

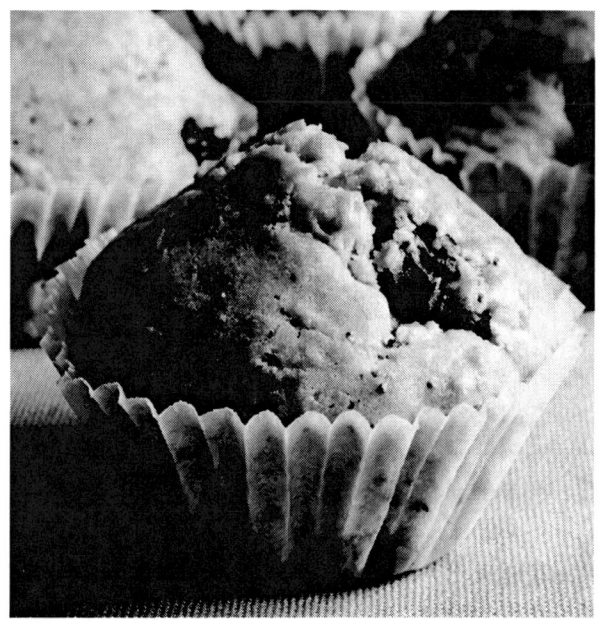

Makes:
12 Servings

Preparation time:
40 minutes

Ingredients:
1 cup fresh washed raspberries
¼ cup coconut oil
¼ cup reduced fat goat cheese
½ cup coconut palm sugar
1 egg
2 cups coconut flour
1 cup skim milk

2 Tbsp. poppy seeds

Directions:
1. Preheat oven to 400 degrees F.

2. Grease 12 muffin tins or plate the paper liners in each of them, your choice.

3. Make sure after washing the raspberries that you drain them really well.

4. Mix together the goat cheese you left room temperature so it is nice and soft with the coconut toil. You can use an electric mixer to make sure it gets smoother.

5. Add the egg and then the milk and gradually the coconut flour and coconut palm sugar as well. Continue mixing.

6. Finally add the raspberries and the poppy seeds. Mix gently and pour the batter into each muffin tin.

7. Bake for a little less than 30 minutes.

Nutrition Information per serving: 150 Calories, 6 g total fat, 20 mg cholesterol, 240 mg sodium, **5.5 g carbonates (sugars),** 1g fiber, and 4g protein.

DELICIOUS DIP FOR YOUR FAVORITE FRUITS

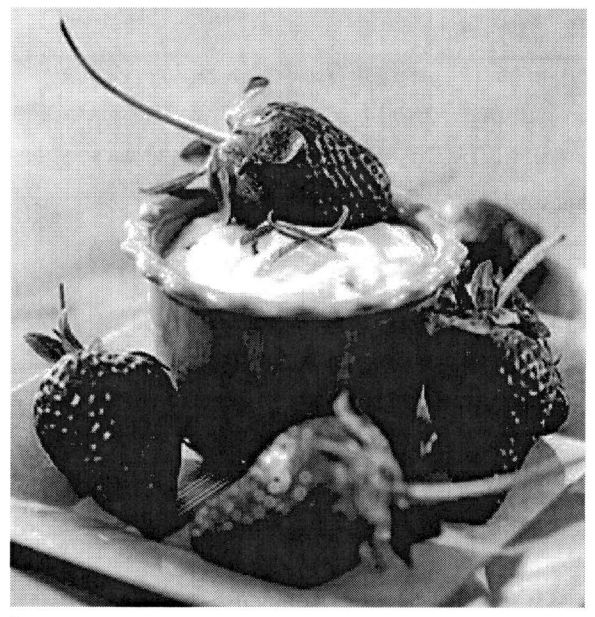

Makes:
8 Servings

Preparation time:
10 minutes

Ingredients:
2 cups fat free sour cream
2 Tbsp. Manuka honey
1 Tbsp. orange zest
2 Tbsp. no sugar added orange juice
Fresh fruits to serve with (strawberries, cherries or other)

Directions:
1. Mix the orange juice, orange zest, sour cream and honey together and refrigerate until ready to serve in a tightly closed container.

2. Prepare the fresh fruits by washing them and cutting them the size you want. This dip could easily be served with pieces of mellow such as honeydew or cantaloupe as well.

Nutrition Information per serving: 48 Calories, 1.2 g total fat, 63mg cholesterol, 41 mg sodium, **10 g carbonates (sugars),** 1g fiber, and 1g protein.

SWEET POTATOES CASSEROLE

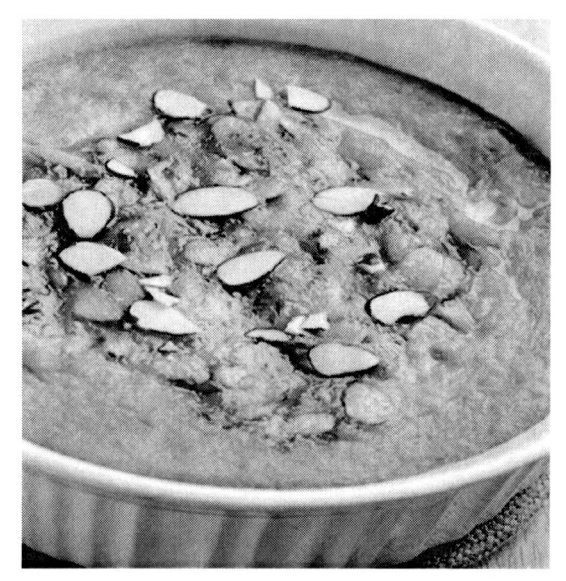

Makes:
8 Servings

Preparation time:
1 hour

Ingredients:
4 large peeled sweet potatoes
¼ cup coconut cream
2 eggs
1 tsp. vanilla extract
½ tsp. cinnamon
½ tsp. nutmeg
½ cup coconut palm sugar
¼ cup coconut oil (room temperature)
¼ cup sugarcane juice
¼ chopped walnuts

1/3 cup coconut flour
3 Tbsp. quinoa flour
Pinch salt

Directions:
1. Preheat oven to 375 degrees F.

2. Prepare a large baking dish by greasing it slightly with coconut oil.

3. Boil some water in large saucepan and after dicing the sweet potatoes, cook them for 20 minutes or until tender.

4. Mash the potatoes once cooked and add the coconut oil, salt, eggs, vanilla, cinnamon, nutmeg and coconut palm sugar.

5. Transfer the mixture into the baking dish.

6. In a separate mixing bowl, mix the sugarcane juice, salt, quinoa flour and coconut flour. Sprinkle the sweet potatoes with the flour mixture.

7. Bake for about 30 minutes and serve warm.

Nutrition Information per serving: 230 Calories, 7 g total fat, 65 mg cholesterol, 150 mg sodium, **36g carbonates (sugars),** 2g fiber, and 5g protein.

DRIED CRANBERRIES AND WALNUTS SCONES

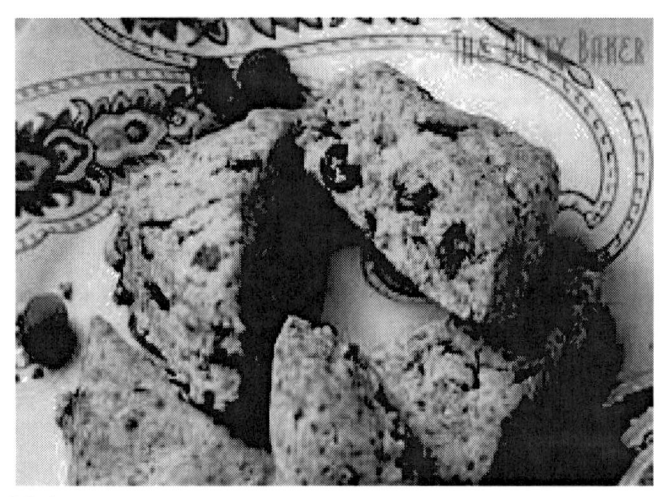

Makes:
12 Servings

Preparation time:
45 minutes

Ingredients:
2 eggs
1/3 cup walnut oil
1 cup pure Stevia
3/4 cup skim milk
½ tsp. vanilla extract
2 cups quinoa flour
1 cup fresh cranberries
¼ cup chopped walnuts
½ tsp. baking soda
½ tsp. baking powder
2 Tbsp. Manuka honey

Directions:
1. Spray with non-stick baking oil the muffin tins. Set aside.

2. Preheat oven at 375 degrees F.

3. Whisk the eggs, walnut oil vanilla, and milk together in a large mixing bowl.

4. In a different bowl mix the dry ingredients: baking powder, baking soda, quinoa flour.

5. Combine both mixtures together next and also add the cranberries, the nuts and the honey. Mix again well.

6. Pour the batter in the muffin tins, it should fill about 10-12. Bake for about 20 minutes or so.

Nutrition Information per serving: 210 Calories, 7 g total fat, 20 mg cholesterol, 130 mg sodium, **33 g carbonates (sugars),** 1g fiber, and 5g protein.

BANANA AND ALMOND BUTTER SMOOTHIE

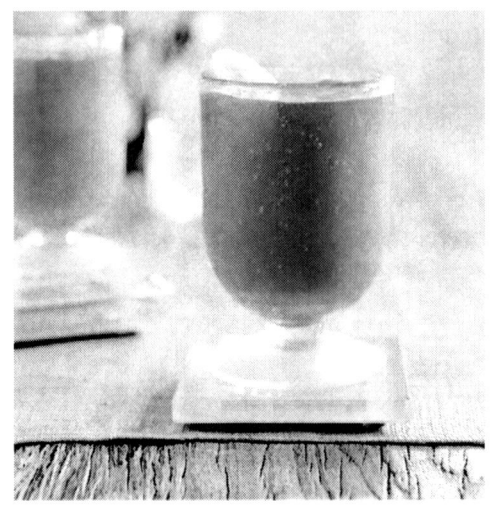

Makes:
4 Servings

Preparation time:
5-8 minutes

Ingredients:
1 small sliced ripe banana
1/2 cup nonfat sour cream
3 Tbsp. almond butter
3 Tbsp. Manuka honey
1 large ripe and sliced banana
Some ice

Directions:

1. Simply blend all ingredients in your high speed blender. Add as much ice as you like in a smoothie.

2. Pour your smoothie in a tall glass and enjoy!

Nutrition Information per serving: 120 Calories, 4 g total fat, 0 mg cholesterol, 100 mg sodium, **16 g carbonates (sugars),** 1g fiber, and 6g protein.

CRISPY BREAKFAST

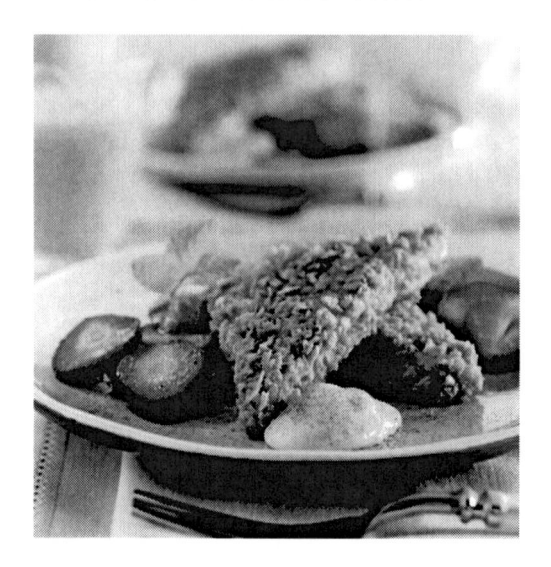

Makes:
6 Servings

Preparation time:
20 minutes

Ingredients:
6 slices bread (made with quinoa flour)
2 cups unsweetened shredded coconut
2 cups coconut flour
1 Tbsp. ground cinnamon
4 large eggs
1 Tsp. almond extract
½ cup coconut palm sugar
1 ½ cup coconut cream
Optional: fruits on the side

Directions:
1. Preheat oven to 375 degrees F.

2. Combine coconut cream, coconut palm sugar, eggs, and almond extract. Whisk well together.

3. In a mixing bowl, mix the dry ingredients (coconut flour, shredded coconut, cinnamon).

4. Cut the slices into triangles or squares.

5. Dip bread pieces into the coconut cream mixture; and then in the flour mixture.

6. Place on a greased baking sheet and bake for about 10 minutes.

7. You can serve it with a diabetic friendly dip and fresh fruits.

Nutrition Information per serving: 300 Calories, 9 g total fat, 155 mg cholesterol, 460 mg sodium, **27 g carbonates (sugars),** 3g fiber, and 12g protein.

YOGOURT DIP

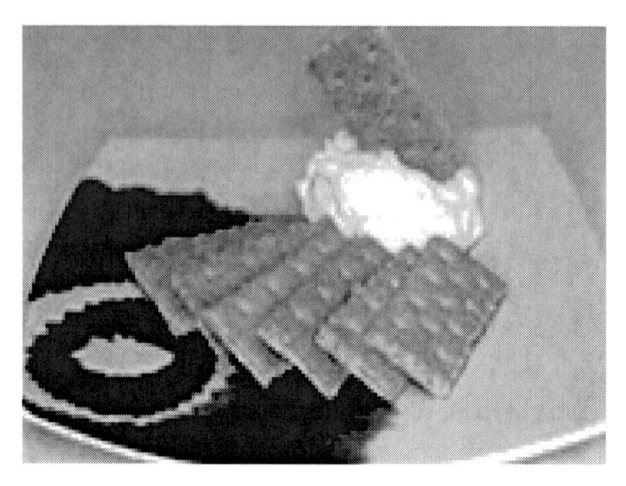

Makes:
12 Servings

Preparation time:
10 minutes

Ingredients:
½ cup low-fat sugar free vanilla yoghurt
½ cup sugar free whipped cream
1 Tbsp. sugarcane juice
Serve with fresh fruits instead of crackers if you can

Directions:
1. Put the yogurt, whipped topping, and sugarcane juice in the blender.

2. You will activate until you are left with a very smooth dip.

3. Serve with your favorite fruits.

Nutrition Information per serving: 100 Calories, 1.5 g total fat, 5 mg cholesterol, 95 mg sodium, **16 g carbonates (sugars),** 1.g fiber, 3g protein.

THE SMOOTHIEST PIE

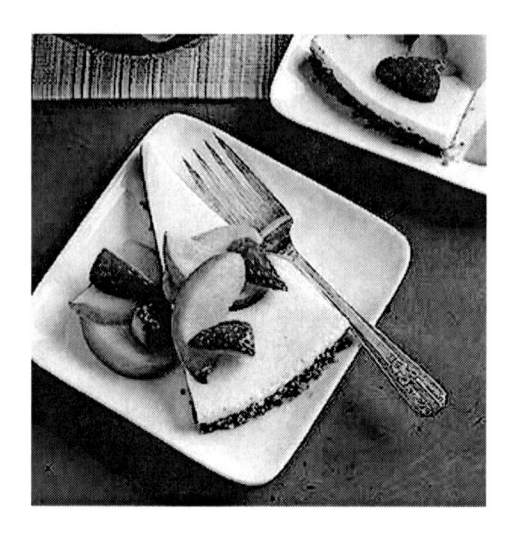

Makes:
12 Servings

Preparation time:
25 minutes

Ingredients:
2 cups fresh sliced peaches or in can (make sure then they are sugar free)
½ cup fresh pitted cherries (cut in halves)
1 cup almond flour
2 Tbsp. pure Stevia
1 envelope unflavored gelatin
½ cup skim milk
1 tsp. almond extract
1 cup sugar free marshmallow cream
¼ cup melted gee butter
Coconut oil to grease

Directions:
1. Preheat oven to 375 degrees F.
2. Prepare the crust first by mixing the almond flour, stevia in a bowl. Add the melted butter and mix well.
3. In a previously greased with coconut oil pie dish, press firmly the crust. Bake for 10 minutes.
4. Meanwhile, prepare the pie filling by mixing the marshmallow cream, milk and unflavored gelatin.
5. Pour the pie filling into the pie crust (when completed cooled down) and refrigerate for a few hours.
6. Decorate with peaches and cherries.

Nutrition Information per serving: 170 Calories, 7 g total fat, 18 mg cholesterol, 126 mg sodium, **24 g carbonates (sugars),** 1g fiber, and 3g protein.

DRIED FRUITS AND NUTS YUMMY SQUARES

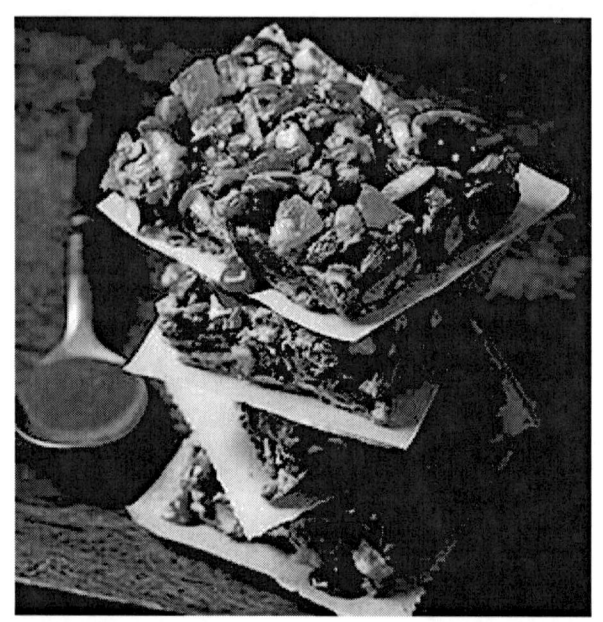

Makes:
12 Servings

Preparation time:
1.5 hour

Ingredients:
Nonstick cooking spray (coconut oil if you can)
3 Tbsp. gee butter
3-4 cups quinoa flour small pretzels (broken in small pieces)
¾ cups dried pineapple pieces
1 cup sunflower seeds
½ cup coconut flour
2 Tbsp. sugarcane juice

3 Tbsp. sugar free caramel sauce
Pinch salt

Directions:
1. In a large baking dish, place parchment paper and let some edges fall over.

2. Melt the butter first in a saucepan on medium heat, stir in the sugar can juice and caramel and mix very well. Wait until it becomes thicker before removing from heat.

3. Stir in the pretzels pieces, sunflower seeds, dried pineapple, coconut flour, and mix very well.

4. It will be sticky, but go ahead and press the mixture into the dish you set aside previously and refrigerator for an hour.

5. Remove from the refrigerator and cut into squares or rectangles. Place the squares into a hermetically sealed container.

6. Eat only one at a time, if you can!

Nutrition Information per serving: 170 Calories, 8.5 g total fat, 5 mg cholesterol, 183 mg sodium, **29 g carbonates (sugars),** 1g fiber, and 4g protein.

VANILLA WARM BEVERAGE

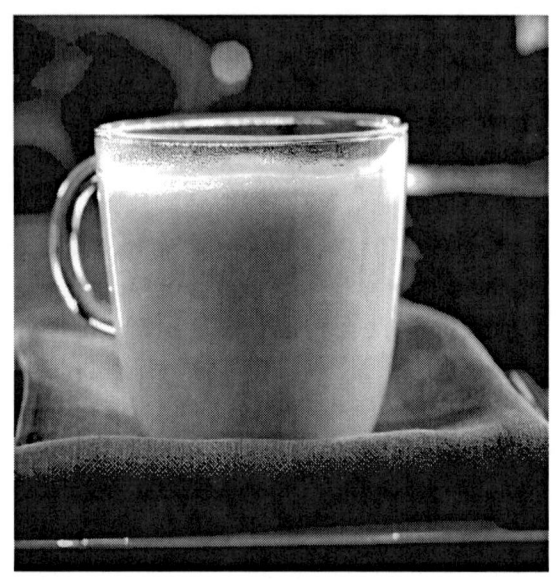

Makes:
1 serving

Preparation time:
12 minutes

Ingredients:
3/4 cup unsweetened almond milk
2 Tbsp. coconut palm sugar
1/4 tsp. almond extract

Directions:
1. Serving a warm and healthy glad of sweet milk is always welcome, especially on a cold day perhaps.

2. Simply combine all ingredients in small saucepan on low heat.

3. Once it's warm enough, transfer into a cup and enjoy!

Nutrition Information per serving: 2 Calories, 8.5 g total fat, 6 mg cholesterol, 95 mg sodium, **9 g carbonates (sugars),** 1g fiber, and 6g protein.

MELON SALAD

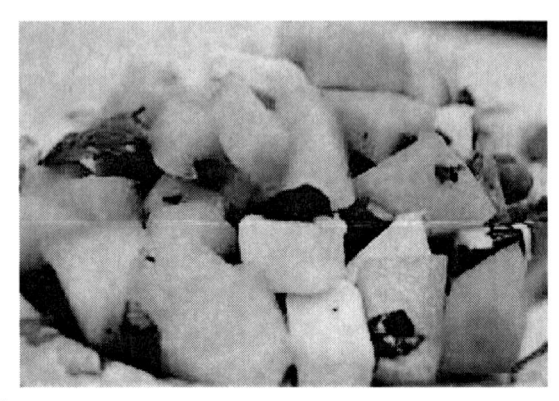

Makes:
8 Servings

Preparation time:
10 minutes

Ingredients:
1 small cantaloupe (peeled and diced)
1 cup watermelon
1 cup diced pineapple
1 Tbsp. lemon juice
1 Tbsp. lime juice
¼ cup Manuka honey
Few chopped finely mint leaves

Directions:
1. Mix the lime and lemon juice with the honey in a small bowl.

2. Prepare all the fruits by cutting them in the size you prefer in a large bowl.

3. Add the citrus juice and honey to the fruits and the mint leaves. Stir well.

4. Serve cold.

Nutrition Information per serving: 80 Calories, 0 g total fat, 0 mg cholesterol, 61 mg sodium, **19 g carbonates (sugars),** 1g fiber, and 1g protein.

GINGERBREAD TASTY LOAF

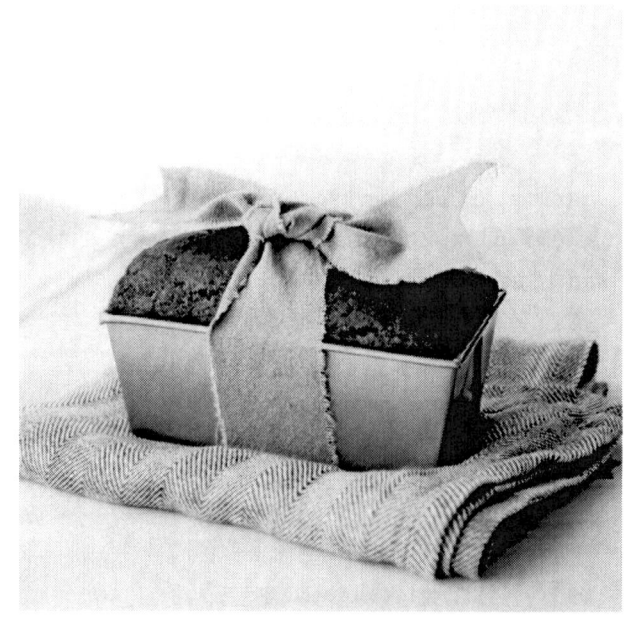

Makes:
12-18 Servings

Preparation time:
1 hour

Ingredients:
2 cups unsweetened applesauce
¾ cup sugarcane juice
1/3 cup coconut oil
3 egg whites
1 cup pure Stevia
1 cups quinoa flour
1 Tbsp. baking soda
1 tsp. baking powder

Pinch salt
1 tsp. ginger
1 tsp. nutmeg
1 tsp. cinnamon

Directions:
1. Preheat oven to 350 degrees F.

2. In a large mixing bowl, combine the sugarcane juice, coconut oil and egg whites. Mix very well.

3. In a separate bowl, combine the dry ingredients (baking powder, baking soda, flour and all spices).

4. Combine the wet and dry mixture, mix well.

5. Finally, add the applesauce to the mixture and stir.

6. You should be able to pour the bread batter in a previously greased baking dish (loaf dish).

7. Bake the bread for about 50 minutes and serve warm or cold.

Nutrition Information per serving: 180 Calories, 5 g total fat, 35 mg cholesterol, 240 mg sodium, **28.5 g carbonates (sugars),** 1g fiber, and 3g protein.

MY FAVORITE PEANUT BUTTER COOKIES

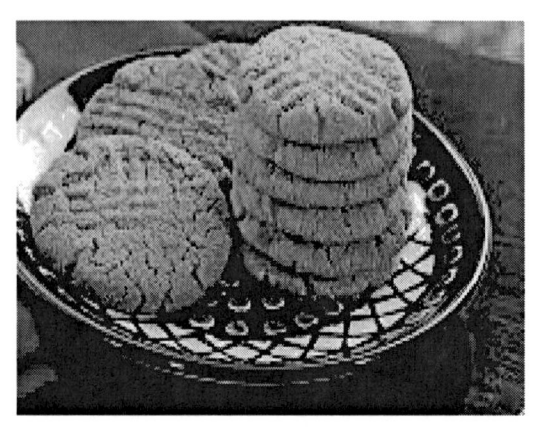

Makes:

16 Servings

Preparation time:

15 minutes

Ingredients:

1/2 cup coconut palm sugar

3 Tbsp. Manuka honey

5 Tbsp. coconut toil (room temperature)

¼ cup creamy no sugar added peanut butter

2 eggs

1 tsp. vanilla

1 3/2 cup almond flour

1/2 tsp. baking soda

Pinch salt

Directions:
1. Preheat oven to 375 degrees F.

2. In a large mixing bowl, go ahead and combine the honey, coconut oil, eggs, vanilla and peanut butter. You should obtain a smooth mixture.

3. Separately first, mix the flour, baking soda, salt and coconut palm sugar.

4. Combine the dry mixture to the wet one and mix again very well.

5. You now have you peanut butter cookies batter.

6. Drop about one teaspoon of the batter at a time on the baking sheet.

7. You should be able to make about 16-20 cookies.

8. Bake for about 10-12 minutes.

9. Enjoy with a glass of skim milk or with black coffee.

Nutrition Information per serving: 60 Calories, 20 g total fat, 0 mg cholesterol, 65 mg sodium, **9 g carbonates (sugars),** 0g fiber, and 1g protein.

A LITTLE SOMETHING TO TOP OFF A FRUIT SALAD

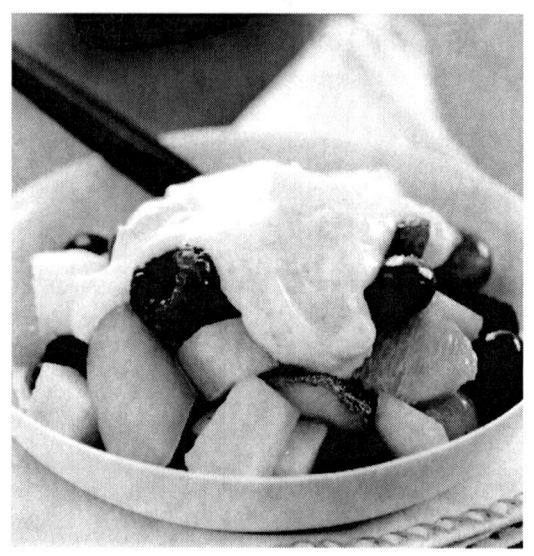

Makes:
6 Servings

Preparation time:
20 minutes

Ingredients:
1 cup fresh sliced strawberries
1 cup fresh raspberries
1 cup fresh blueberries
1 cup diced cantaloupe
1 cup diced Granny smith apple (I prefer to leave the peel on)
2 Tbsp. lime juice

Yoghurt dip

1 Tbsp. pumpkin pie spice

2 cups low fat sugar free plain yoghurt

2 Tbsp. Manuka honey

Directions:

1. Prepare all the fresh fruits in a large bowl. Drizzle the little lime juice on the fresh fruits to make sure no one turn brownish.

2. Prepare the yoghurt dip in a separate bowl by missing the yoghurt, pumpkin spice and honey.

3. Serve anytime of the year, it is always so refreshing and delicious!

Nutrition Information per serving: 170 Calories, 2 g total fat, 5mg cholesterol, 35 mg sodium, **39 g carbonates (sugars),** 1g fiber, and 7g protein.

APPLE AND RAISINS TOPPING

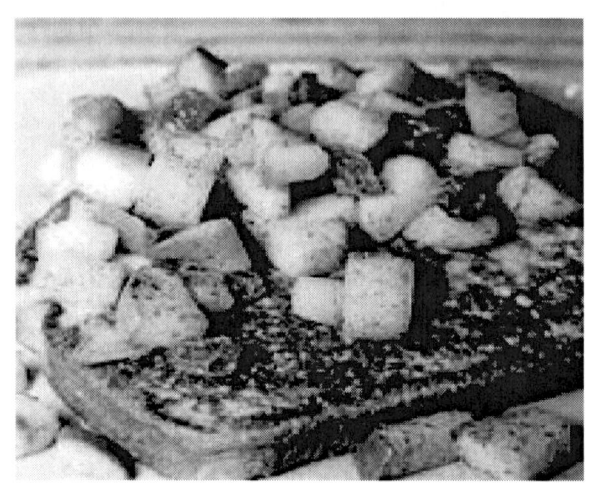

Makes:
6 Servings

Preparation time:
12 minutes

Ingredients:
3 diced red delicious apple or Gala, your choice
2 Tbsp. gee butter
3 Tbsp. dried raisins
1/2 tsp. ground cinnamon
1/2 Tsp. minced fresh ginger

Directions:
1. After getting all ingredients ready, warm up the butter in the skillet and sautéed the apples with the spices and dried raisins.

2. Remember, this is a topping you can use on applesauce, on your diabetic friendly French toasts or pancakes. Just delicious!

Nutrition Information per serving: 203 Calories, 2.1 g total fat, 62 mg cholesterol, 189 mg sodium, **41 g carbonates (sugars),** 1.2g fiber, and 6g protein.

FUN POPSICLES

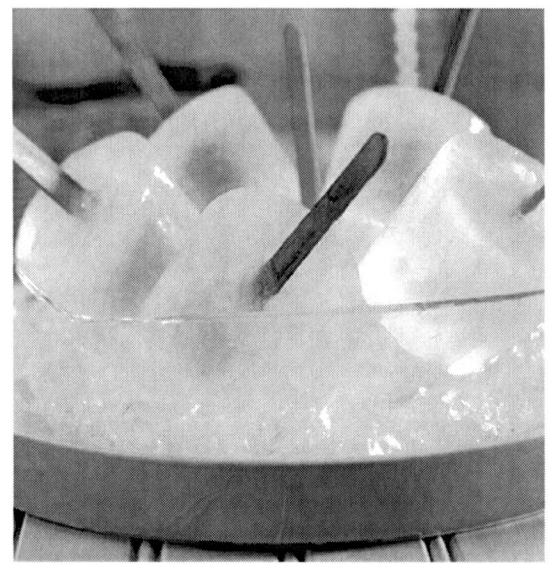

Makes:
10-12 Servings

Preparation time:
15 minutes

Ingredients:
1 package of unsweetened drink mix (lemonade flavor is great)
1 cup pure Stevia
2 quarts cold water
12-16 popsicles sticks- molds

Directions:

1. Mix the lemonade mix and the water in a large pitcher. Mix well and add also the Stevia. Mix again.

2. Pour the drink mixture into your popsicles molds and freeze until they are frozen and hard.

3. Lick away!

Nutrition Information per serving: 85 Calories, 0 g total fat, 0 mg cholesterol, 45 mg sodium, **7 g carbonates (sugars),** 0.1g fiber, and 0.5g protein.

VERY BERRIES SMOOTHIE

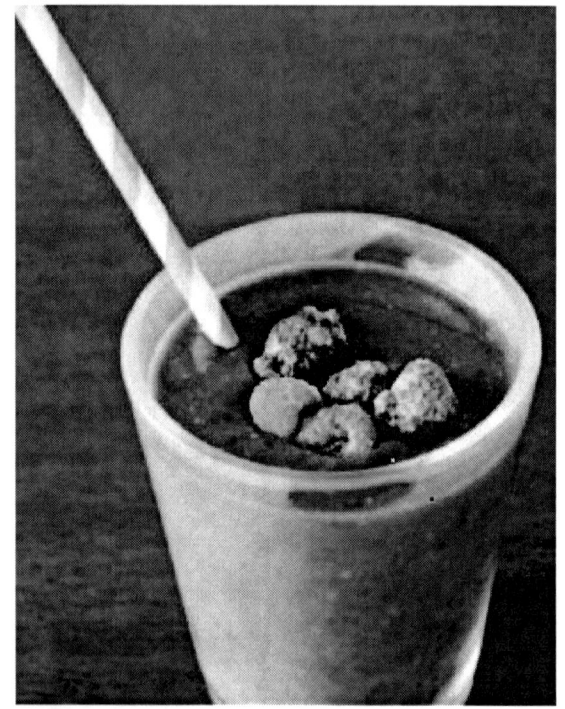

Makes:
2 Servings

Preparation time:
10 minutes

Ingredients:
2 cups unsweetened vanilla cashew milk
1 Tbsp. Manuka honey
1/2 cup fresh raspberries
1/2 cup fresh blueberries
1 Tbsp. lemon juice

Directions:
1. Blend all ingredients in your high speed blender until the texture is smooth as it should be.

2. Pour in a tall glass. Save a few fresh fruits on the side to decorate your smoothie with.

Nutrition Information per serving: 152 Calories, 8.5 g total fat, 6 mg cholesterol, 61 mg sodium, **17.5 g carbonates (sugars),** 1g fiber, and 3.5g protein.

YOUR KID'S LUNCH BOX

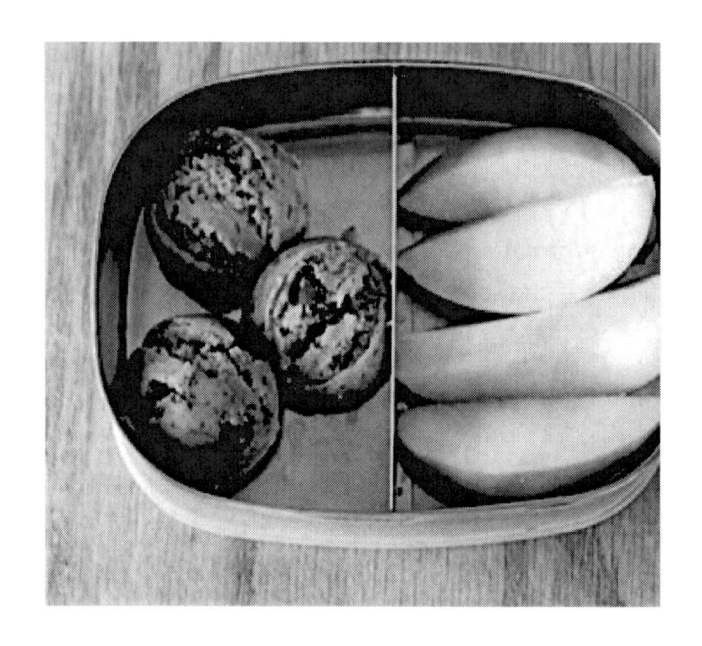

Makes:
12-14 Servings

Preparation time:
15 minutes

Ingredients:

½ cup creamy almond butter

½ tsp. almond extract

1 Tbsp. sugarcane juice

¼ cup almond flour

3 Tbsp. flax seeds

Pinch salt

¼ cup carob chips

Directions:

1. Your kids love cookies of course, but if you have a child who is diabetic, it is concern and you should be careful about what you pack in their lunch for sure.

2. These cookies are safe and your kids will love them.

3. In a mixing bowl, combine the almond butter, sugarcane juice, almond extract and mix well.

4. In a different bowl combine the dry ingredients: salt, flaxseeds and almond flour. Then mix both the dry and wet ingredients together.

5. Use your hands to mix well. Finally add the carob chips and mix again. Form the cookies dough drops- portions. Choose the size depending on the age and appetite of your children.

6. Refrigerate the dough for at least 45 minutes before serving.

Nutrition Information per serving: 152 Calories, 8.5 g total fat, 6 mg cholesterol, 61 mg sodium, **17.5 g carbonates (sugars),** 1g fiber, and 3.5g protein.

APPLE CRUMBLES FOR EVERYONE

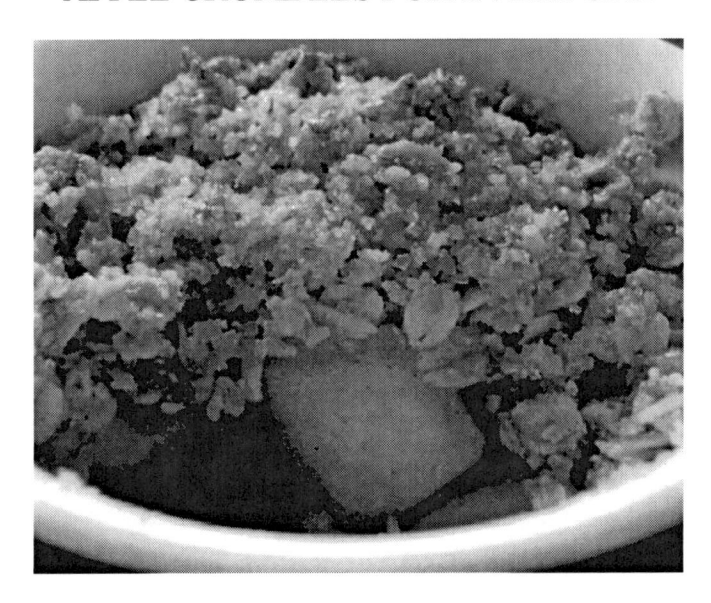

Makes: 6 Servings

Prep: 50 minutes

Ingredients:
1/3 cup coconut flour
3 Tbsp. coconut oil
3 Tbsp. coconut palm sugar
3 Tbsp. water
1 -1.5 pound of your favorite apples: Granny Smith, Gala or Red delicious)

Directions:
1. Preheat oven to 300 degrees F.

2. In a mixing bowl, combine the flour and the room temperature coconut oil, it should be crumbly. Add the coconut palm sugar and mix some more. Set aside.

3. Slice the apples in thin slices or cubes as you wish and place them evenly in a rectangle baking dish.

4. I use also coconut oil to grease the dish. Sprinkle the coconut mixture on top and place in the oven.

5. Bake for about 40 minutes. Serve warm with sugar whipped cream

Nutrition Information per serving: 320 Calories, 5.2 g total fat, 0 mg cholesterol, 201 mg sodium, **25.2 g carbonates (sugars),** 1.2.g fiber, 7g protein.

DELICIOUS ANYTIME BITES

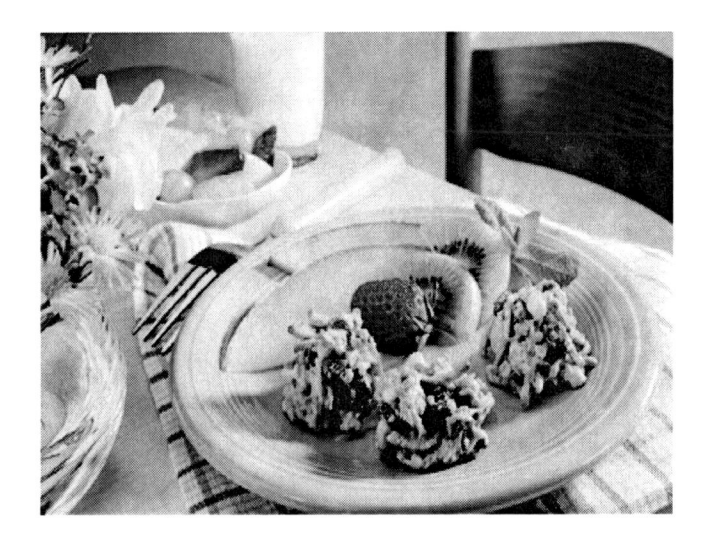

Makes:
24 Servings

Preparation time:
25 minutes

Ingredients:
2 cups gluten free and sugar free cereals (similar to cornflakes)
½ cup almond flour
3/4cup creamy sugar free peanut butter
1 large egg
1 cup pure Stevia
2 tbsp. Vanilla
½ cup golden dried raisins
'

Directions:

1. Preheat oven to 375 degrees F.

2. In a large bowl, mix the chosen cereals, stevia almond flour and raisins.

3. In a different bowl, mix the peanut butter, egg, vanilla and ginger.

4. Pour the second mixture over the first over and combine gently.

5. After greased a baking sheet or 2, drop about a tablespoon of the mixture at a time.

6. Bake for about 10-12 minutes. Set aside and store in an airtight container when cooled down.

Nutrition Information per serving: 60 Calories, 7 g total fat, 0 mg cholesterol, 42 mg sodium, **8g carbonates (sugars),**1.2g fiber, and 2g protein.

MIXED APPLE SAUCE

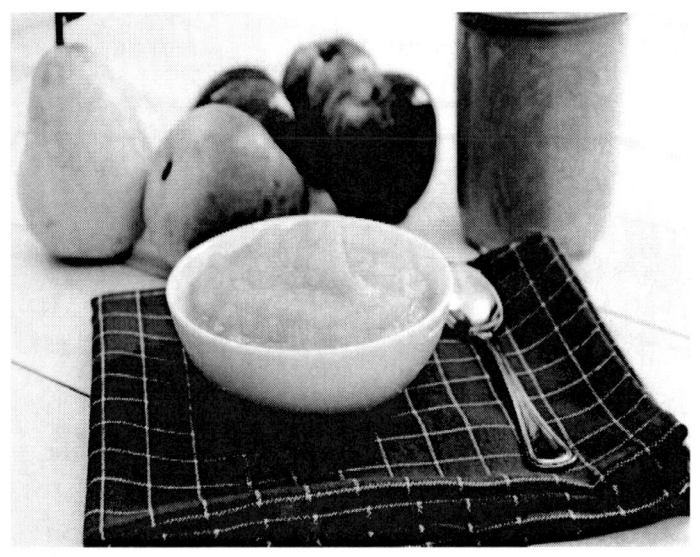

Makes:
4 Servings

Preparation time:
35 minutes

Ingredients:
2 ripe Bartlett pears
2 apples (your choice)
2 Tbsp. orange juice
1 Tbsp. lemon juice
2 Tbsp. Manuka honey
½ tsp. nutmeg
½ tsp. cinnamon

Directions:

1. Prepare the fruits. Cut them in small pieces and place all of them in a medium saucepan.

2. Add the orange and lemon juice, honey and spices. Bring to boil. If needed add a little water. When boiling, reduce to low heat and cook for 25 minutes.

3. You can serve the sauce as is with fruits chunks or you can also place it in the blender and reduce it in puree. That is totally your choice.

Nutrition Information per serving: 95 Calories, 2 g total fat, 0 mg cholesterol, 1mg sodium, **21 g carbonates (sugars),**2g fiber, and 1g protein.

"BLUE" GRANITA

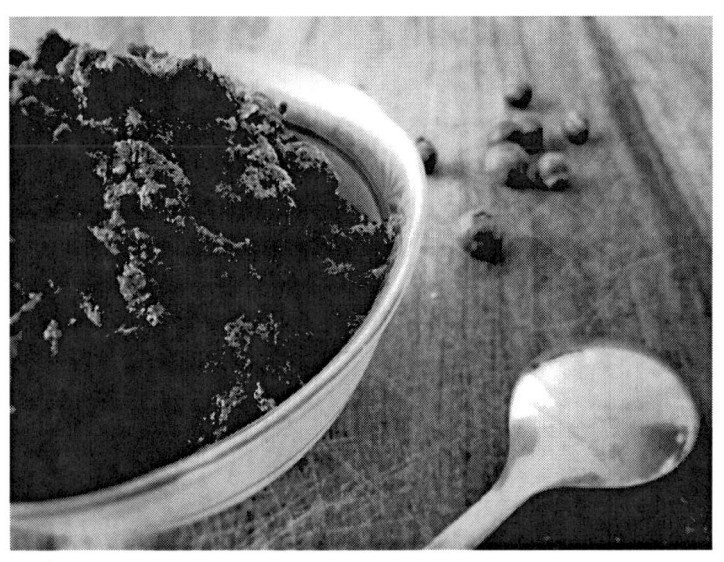

Makes:
4 Servings

Preparation time:
15 minutes

Ingredients:
1 1/4 cups tab water
2 cups fresh blueberries
¼ cup coconut palm sugar
1 Tbsp. sugar free cranberry juice
½ Tbsp. minced fresh mint leaves

Directions:
1. Place all ingredients, except the mint leaves in your high speed blender. Blend until the mixture is fine.

2. Place the mixture into a baking dish of your choice, knowing it will need to fit in your freezer for an hour or so.

3. Cover the dish with foil and freeze for about 30 minutes at a time. Remove from freezer, crush with fork each time and place back in the freezer.

4. Proceed with this step about 5 or 6 time.

5. Serve in your favorite bowls or cups when ready and eta immediately.

Nutrition Information per serving: 50 Calories, 7 g total fat, 0 mg cholesterol, 5 mg sodium, **12g carbonates (sugars),** 2g fiber, and 1g protein.

ORANGE MUFFINS

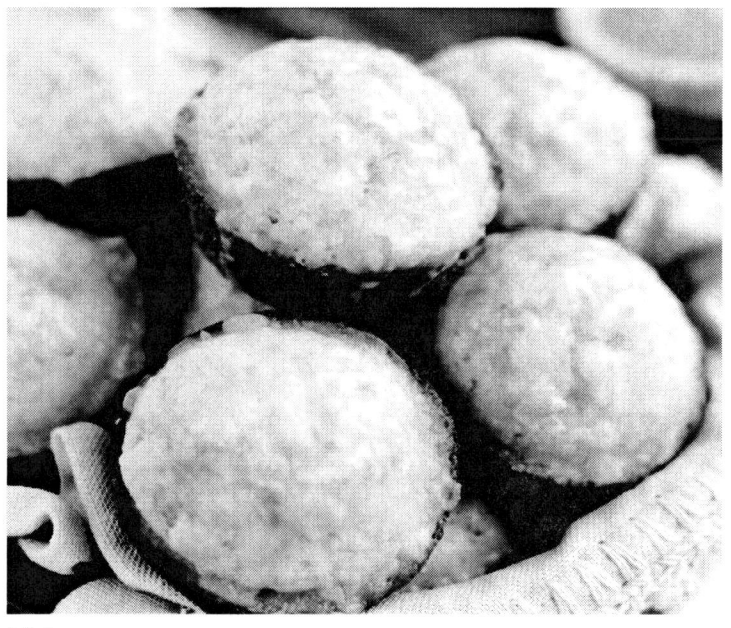

Makes:
12 Servings

Preparation time:
30 minutes

Ingredients:
2 cups quinoa flour
1 cup pure stevia
1 tsp. baking powder
Pinch salt
1 cup orange juice (no sugar added)
1 Tbsp. lemon juice
4 Tbsp. coconut oil
1 large egg

1 tsp. orange zest
1 tsp. lemon zest

Directions:
1. Preheat oven to 350 degrees F.

2. Spray with non-stick cooking spray your muffins tins/. Set aside.

3. In a large bowl, mix all dry ingredients: flour, salt, Stevia, baking powder.

4. In a different bowl, mix the wet ingredients: orange juice, lemon juice, coconut oil, egg and orang, lemon zests.

5. Combine both mixtures and mix well but don't overdo it.

6. Pour the muffin batter evenly in each muffin tin. Bake for about 20 to 25 minutes.

Nutrition Information per serving: 175 Calories, 7 g total fat, 143 mg cholesterol, 18 mg sodium, **26 g carbonates (sugars),** 2g fiber, and 5g protein.

NOT ANOTHER GREEN SMOOTHIE

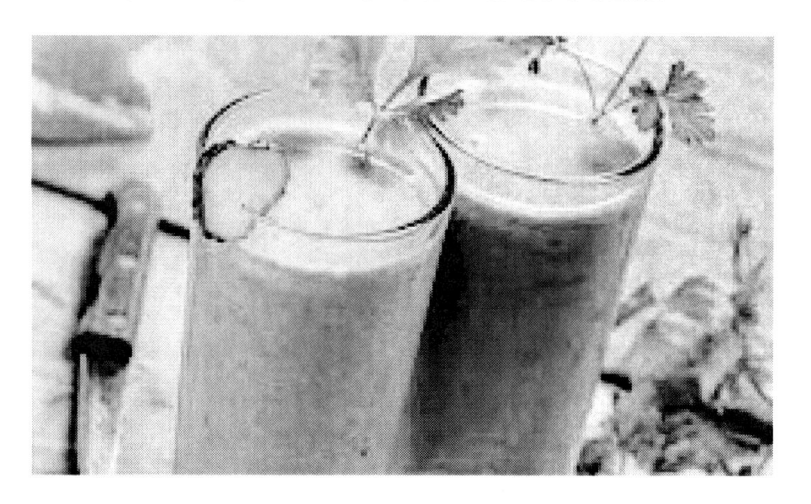

Makes:
2 Servings

Preparation time:
10 minutes

Ingredients:
1 cup unsweetened coconut milk
1 cup baby spinach leaves
2 celery stalk
1 cup strawberries (fresh or frozen)\
½ cup plain Greek yogurt (no sugar added)
½ Tbsp. chia seeds

Directions:
1. Simply blend all ingredients first except the yogurt in your high speed blender.

2. Add the yogurt next and blend again. If you would like, you could add some ice cubes.

3. Serve this green and healthy smoothie in your favorite fancy glass, why not!

Nutrition Information per serving: 90 Calories, 0.5 g total fat, 0 mg cholesterol, 26mg sodium, **17 g carbonates (sugars),** 3g fiber, and 1g protein.

BAKED APPLES

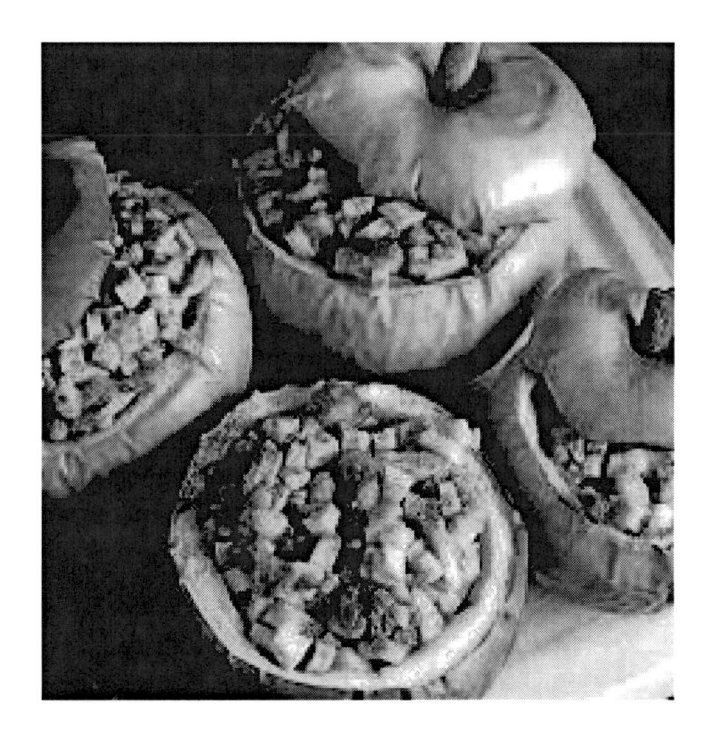

Makes:
8 Servings

Preparation time:
45 minutes

Ingredients:
6-8 apples (depending how many guests or family members you are serving)
1-2 cups water
1 Tbsp. cinnamon
2 Tbsp. orange juice

¼ cup coconut palm sugar
¼ cup coconut flour
2 Tbsp. Manuka honey

Directions:
1. Do not peel the apples. Remove the core from the top, and also the inside of the apple, leaving the bottom to hold up the filling.

2. Keep all the inside of the apples and dice them finely. Add the orange juice to the apples, along with the honey.

3. Place back the apple mixture into each apple "shells".

4. In a small bowl, mix the coconut palm sugar and coconut flour. You will then use it as topping for the apples.

5. Place all apples in a baking dish with the water in the bottom. Bake for about 30 minutes or until apples are fully cooked.

Nutrition Information per serving: 100 Calories, 0.5 g total fat, 0 mg cholesterol, 5mg sodium, **21 g carbonates (sugars),** 4g fiber, and 0g protein.

TOO GOOD TO BE TRUE CANDIES

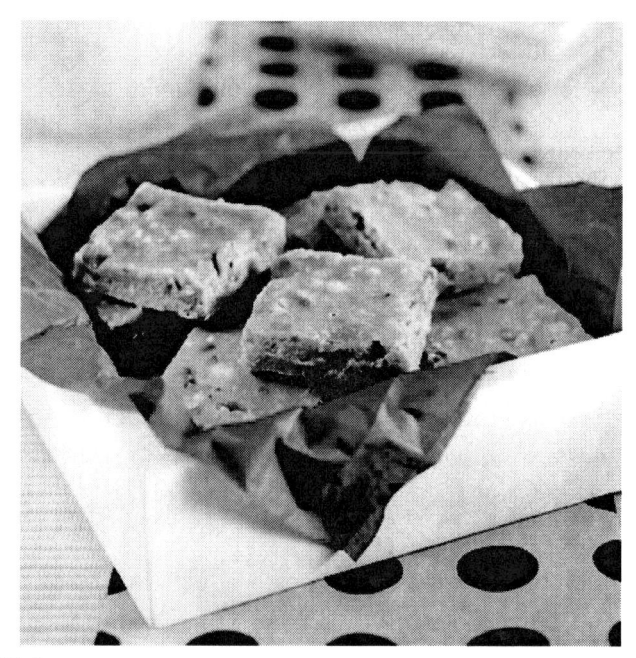

Makes:
16 Servings

Preparation time:
35 minutes

Ingredients:
3/4 cup pure Stevia
1 cup coconut palm sugar
1/3 cup coconut cream
1/3 cup skim milk
2 Tbsp. gee butter
1 tsp. almond extract
1/2 cup chopped pecans and walnut mix

Directions:
Prepare a square baking dish by greasing it. I usually use a little coconut oil.

In a large saucepan, combine the coconut palm sugar, stevia, coconut cream and skim milk, .Bring to boil and once it boils, lower temperature to low. Let it simmer for about 20 minutes.

Add the butter and almond extract and stir only once. Let is cool down naturally.

Add the nuts and stir a few times.

Pour the mixture into the greased dish and set aside. When the candy is completely cooled, cut in squares. If needed, you can refrigerate for a little while to help cutting the candies.

Nutrition Information per serving: 152 Calories, 1.5 g total fat, 6 mg cholesterol, 25 mg sodium, **23 g carbonates (sugars),** 0g fiber, and 1g protein.

THE PERFECT HOLIDAY LOAF

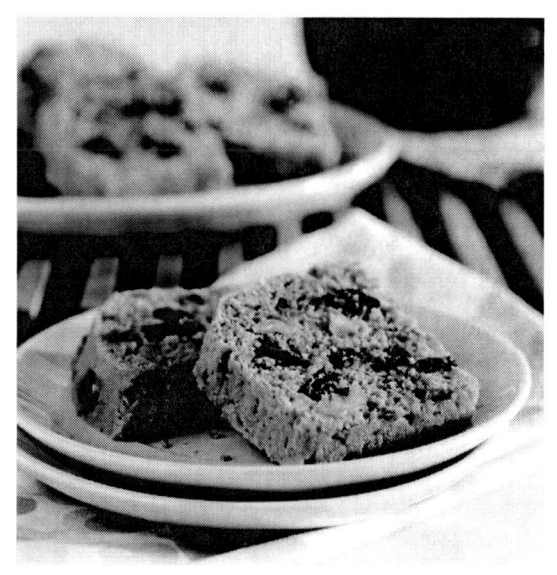

Makes:
12-16 Servings

Preparation time:
45 minutes to 1 hour

Ingredients:
1/3 cup fat free sour cream
2 cups unsweetened pumpkin puree
3 eggs
2 cups quinoa flour
½ cup almond flour
¼ cup walnut oil
¾ cup pure Stevia
2 Tbsp. baking powder
1 Tbsp. Pumpkin pie spice
1 cup dried raisins

Directions:
1. Preheat oven to 350 degrees F.

2. In a large mixing bowl, mix the sour cream, pumpkin puree, eggs and walnut oil.

3. Add next the dry ingredients: quinoa flour, almond flour, Stevia, baking powder and spices. Mix well.

4. Finally add the dried raisins. Mix again and pour this wonderful mixture into a greased loaf pan.

5. Bake for 45-50 minutes. Serve warm or cold.

Nutrition Information per serving: 180 Calories, 6 g total fat, 40 mg cholesterol, 140 mg sodium, **28.5 g carbonates (sugars),** 1.1g fiber, and 5g protein.

PEAR AND HONEY SCONES

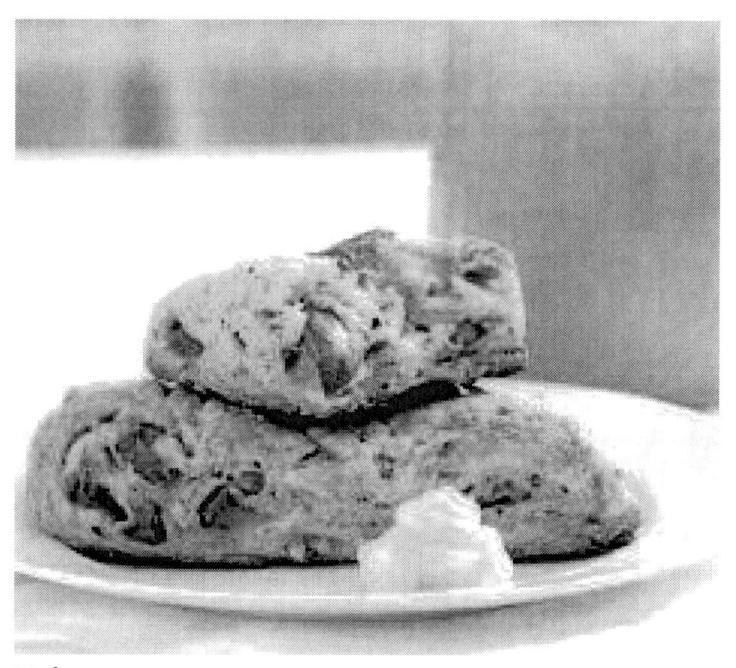

Makes:
10 Servings

Preparation time:
15 minutes

Ingredients:
2 cups coconut flour
Pinch salt
1 Tbsp. baking powder
½ tsp. baking soda
¼ cup flaxseeds
1/3 cup coconut oil
2 chopped finely fresh and ripe pears (peeled)

½ cup skim milk
¼ cup Manuka honey
1 tsp. ground cinnamon

Directions:
1. Preheat oven to 400 degrees F.

2. Combine the dry ingredients first in a large mixing bowl: coconut flour, flaxseeds, baking powder, salt, baking soda.

3. Add the coconut oil (room temperature) gradually, while mixing and then the pears, milk, honey. Mix until the mixture becomes nice and moist.

4. You will be left with nice dough and can roll it into a large circle or square.

5. To prepare the scone shape, cut into 10 wedges and bake on a greased baking sheet for about 20 minutes.

Nutrition Information per serving: 223 Calories, 3.8 g total fat, 0 mg cholesterol, 270 mg sodium, **36 g carbonates (sugars),** 2.1g fiber, and 5g protein.

ANOTHER INTERESTING BROWNIES RECIPE

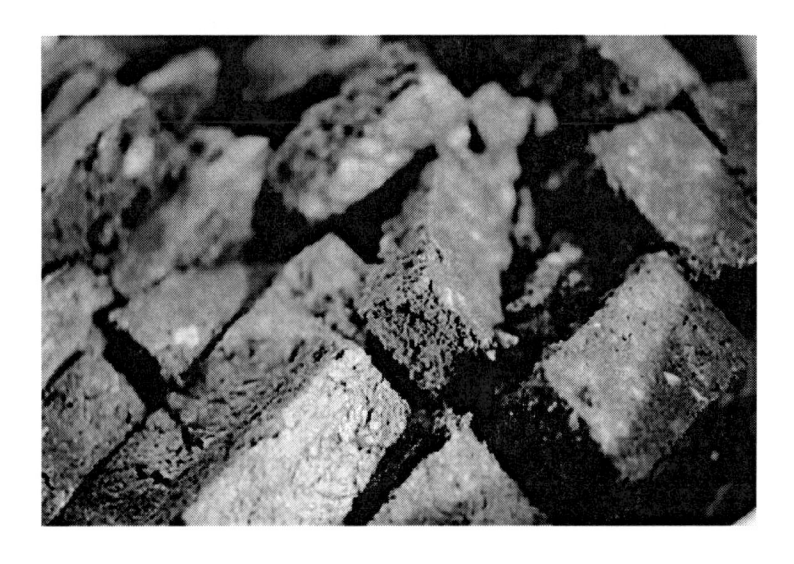

Makes:
16 Servings

Preparation time:
15 minutes

Ingredients:
1/3 cup coconut oil
1/2 cup unsweetened applesauce
1/2 cup unsweetened cocoa powder
1/2 cup coconut palm sugar
1 cup quinoa flour
1 tsp. baking powder
1/2 tsp. baking soda
2 large eggs
1 tsp. vanilla extract

1/4 cup chopped pecans

Directions:
1. Preheat oven to 375 degrees F.

2. Combine the coconut oil, applesauce and cocoa powder. Add the coconut palm sugar and let it dissolved.

3. Also add the eggs and vanilla next and mix well.

4. In a separate bowl, combine together the dry ingredients (quinoa flour, baking soda, baking powder). Add to the first mixture. Mix again.

5. Pour this new batter into the previously greased square baking dish. Sprinkle on the chopped pecans.

6. Bake the brownies for 25 minutes.

7. Cut in squares and enjoy!

Nutrition Information per serving: 165 Calories, 7 g total fat, 101 mg cholesterol, 85 mg sodium, **21 g carbonates (sugars),** 0.2g fiber, and 3g protein.

SWEET POTATO PIE, JUST SWEET ENOUGH

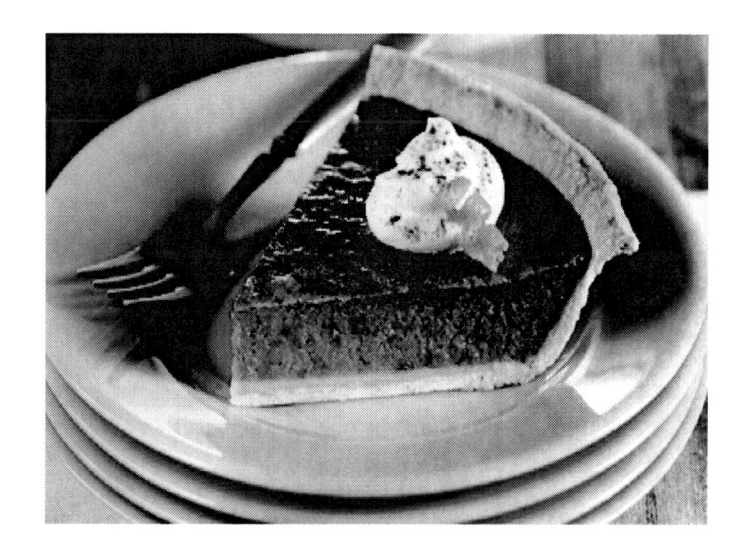

Makes:
8 Servings

Preparation time:
15 minutes

Ingredients:
Diabetic friendly pre-cooked pie crust (look for gluten free and the type of flours you are allowed to eat on your diet, no sugar added, of course)
2 cups mashed sweet potatoes (equivalent to 22 or 3 cooked potatoes)
2 medium eggs
1 cup coconut palm sugar
2 Tbsp. coconut flour
1 Tbsp. Lemon juice

1 tsp. almond extract
½ tsp. ground cloves
½ tsp. cinnamon
1 can coconut milk
Sugar free whipped cream (optional topping)

Directions:
1. Place the cooked sweet potatoes in large mixing bowl; add the coconut palm sugar, lemon juice and blend with your electric mixer until it is smooth.

2. Add next the eggs, almond extract, spices, coconut milk, and coconut flour.

3. Pour this sweet potato mixture into the pie crust and cook for about 40 minutes.

4. Serve warm with whipped cream. Some people prefer to eat it cold or room temperature, that's my preference, for sure.

Nutrition Information per serving: 197 Calories, 67 g total fat, 58 mg cholesterol, 316 mg sodium, **27.5 g carbonates (sugars),** 0.2g fiber, and 7g protein.

DID YOU SAY HEALTHY DONUTS?

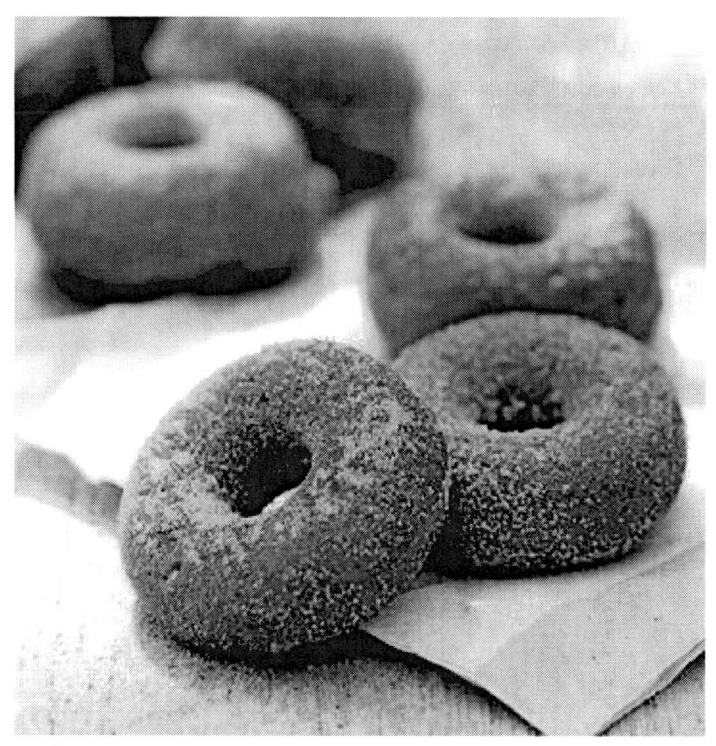

Makes:
12 Servings

Preparation time:
20 minutes

Ingredients:
1 1/4 cups almond or coconut flour (your preference)
1/2 tsp. baking soda
Pinch salt
1/2 cup low fat sour cream
1 egg

1/2 cup pure Stevia
2 Tbsp. coconut oil
1 tsp. vanilla
½ tsp. cinnamon
For optional topping: coconut palm sugar

Directions:
1. Preheat oven to 3 degrees F. As you can tell we are not going to try the donuts, but bake them.

2. You should have a donut pan and you should spray some non-stick baking oil (like coconut oil).

3. In a bowl, combine the chosen flour, baking soda and salt.

4. In a different bowl, mix the sour cream, Stevia, egg, coconut oil and vanilla.

5. Add the wet mixture to the dry and mix until it is al blended.

6. Place batter in the doughnut pan, do not exceed the mold, it will get messy.

7. Sprinkle with the coconut palm sugar.

8. Bake for about 10 minutes, watch it closely.

Nutrition Information per serving: 172 Calories, 4 g total fat, 1 mg cholesterol, 180 mg sodium, **32 g carbonates (sugars),** 2g fiber, and 4g protein.

DIABETIC APPROVED PUMPKIN PIE

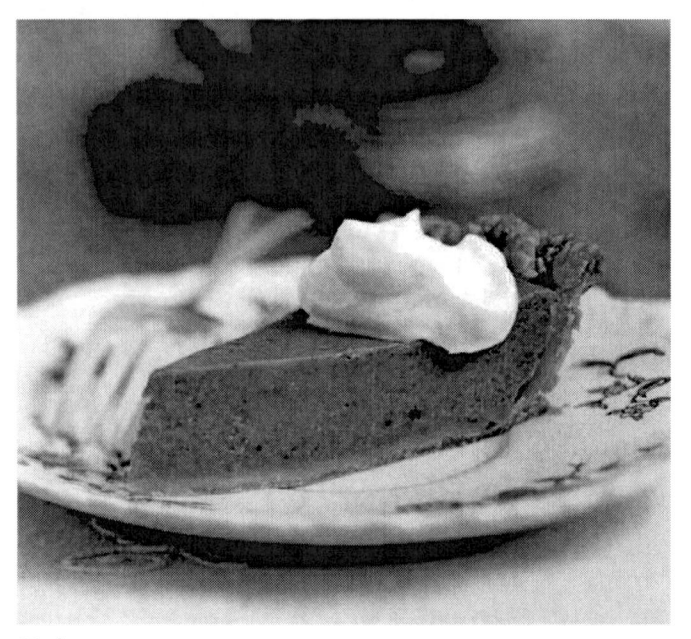

Makes:
8 Servings

Preparation time:
1 hour minimum

Ingredients:
1 diabetic friendly pie crust
1 large unsweetened pumpkin puree
2 egg whites
1 cup almond milk
Pinch salt
½ tsp. ginger
½ tsp. cinnamon
½ tsp. nutmeg

2 Tbsp. sugarcane juice
2 Tbsp. coconut palm sugar

Directions:
1. Preheat oven to 375 degrees F.

2. In a large bowl mix all ingredients. It will make your pie filling. Taste and adjust the seasonings if you like.

3. Pour the filing into the pie crust.

4. Bake in the oven for 50 minutes and serve with a scoop of sugar free whipped cream if you want to.

Nutrition Information per serving: 256 Calories, 3 g total fat, 104 mg cholesterol, 45 mg sodium, **21 g carbonates (sugars),** 0.2g fiber, and 4g protein.

DATES BREAD

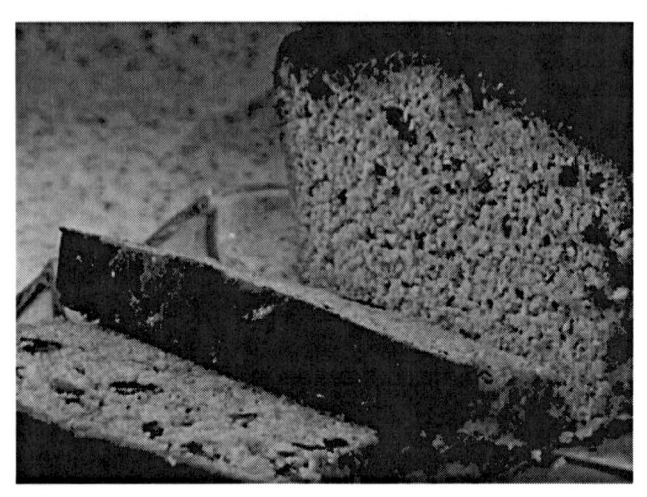

Makes:
12 Servings

Preparation time:
45 minutes

Ingredients:
1/2 cup diced dried dates
½ cup cold water
1 cup almond flour
½ cup quinoa flour
1 tsp. baking powder
1 tsp. nutmeg
1 tsp. cinnamon
Pinch salt
¾ cup coconut palm sugar
½ cup unsweetened almond milk
¼ cup walnut oil
1 large egg

1 tsp. almond extract

Directions:
1. Preheat the oven to 350 degrees F.

2. Prepare a loaf dish by spraying nonstick oil evenly. Set aside.

3. You should place the dates in water in a small saucepan and cook on medium heat for 10-15 minutes, so they get softer. Set aside and let cool down when done.

4. In a medium bowl, mix the almond and quinoa flour, salt, baking powder and spices.

5. In a different bowl, combine the other ingredients, except the dates. Then, combine both mixtures together to get your loaf batter.

6. Add the dates and mix lightly again. Pour the final batter into you're the baking dish and bake in the oven for about 40 minutes.

Nutrition Information per serving: 142 Calories, 5 g total fat, 14 mg cholesterol, 71 mg sodium, **24 g carbonates (sugars),**3g fiber, and 2g protein.

ZUCHINNI CITRUS BREAD

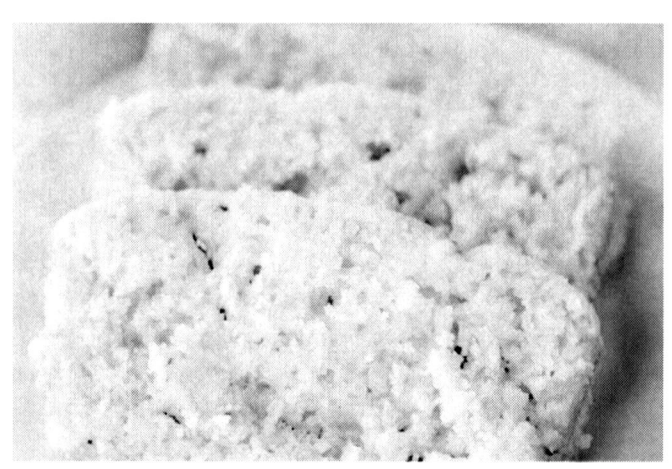

Makes:
10-16 Servings

Preparation time:
1 hour to 1 .5 hour

Ingredients:
1 cup shredded zucchini (peeled)
1 cup almond flour
½ cup coconut flour
½ coconut palm sugar
1 Tbsp. sugarcane juice
Pinch salt
1/3 cup chopped pistachios
1/3 cup coconut oil
1 Tbsp. lime juice
1 tsp. lime zest
½ cup almond milk
2 large eggs
1 tsp. ginger

Directions:
1. Preheat the oven to 350 degrees F.
2. Greased a loaf pan with coconut oil and set aside.
3. In a large mixing bowl, combine the flours, coconut pal sugar, baking soda and stir in the shredded zucchini, pistachios, lime zest, lime juice and ginger.
4. Whisk the eggs, almond milk and coconut oil in s separate bowl and add to the dry mixture, mix again.
5. Pour the batter in the baking dish and bake for about 55 minutes.

Nutrition Information per serving: 122 Calories, 6 g total fat, 24 mg cholesterol, 206 mg sodium, **15 g carbonates (sugars),** 1g fiber, and 2g protein.

MUFFINS FILLED WITH PEACHES

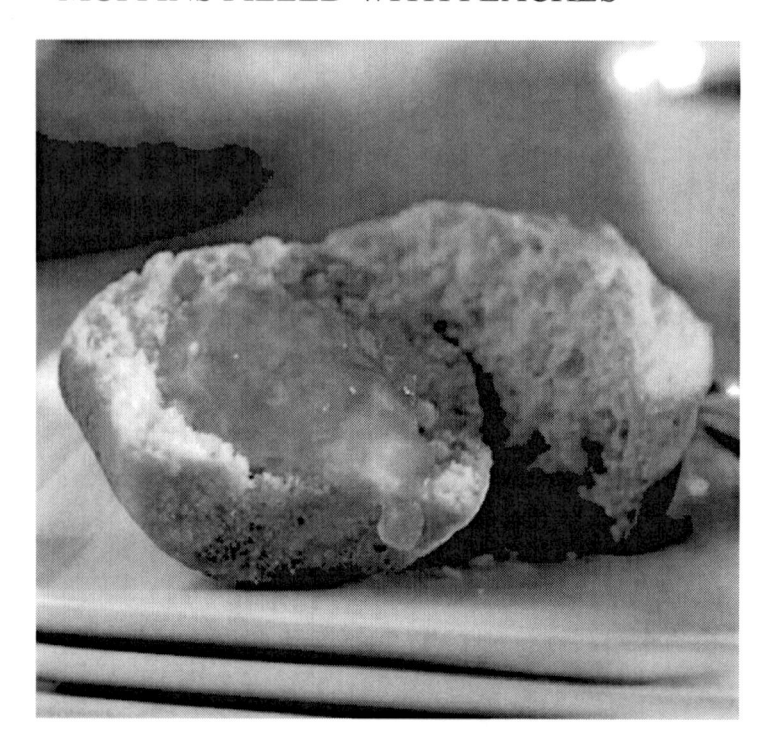

Makes:
8-12 Servings

Preparation time:
45 minutes

Ingredients:
1 cup quinoa flour
¼ cup pure stevia
2 tsp. baking powder
Pinch salt
1 large egg
2 Tbsp. gee butter

2 Tbsp. skim milk
½ cup Peaches sugar free preserve-jam
¼ tsp. vanilla extract

Directions:
1. Preheat oven to 350 degrees F.

2. Coat the muffin tins with spray nonstick cooking oil.

3. In a mixing bowl, combine the flour, the stevia, baking powder and salt.

4. In a separate bowl, whisk the egg, butter and milk. Combine both mixtures, add the almond extract after and mix again.

5. Pour the batter into the muffin tins and bake for about 22-25 minutes.

Nutrition Information per serving: 150 Calories, 17 g total fat, 35 mg cholesterol, 190 mg sodium, **24 g carbonates (sugars),** 0g fiber, and 3g protein.

PEANUT BUTTER DELIGHT

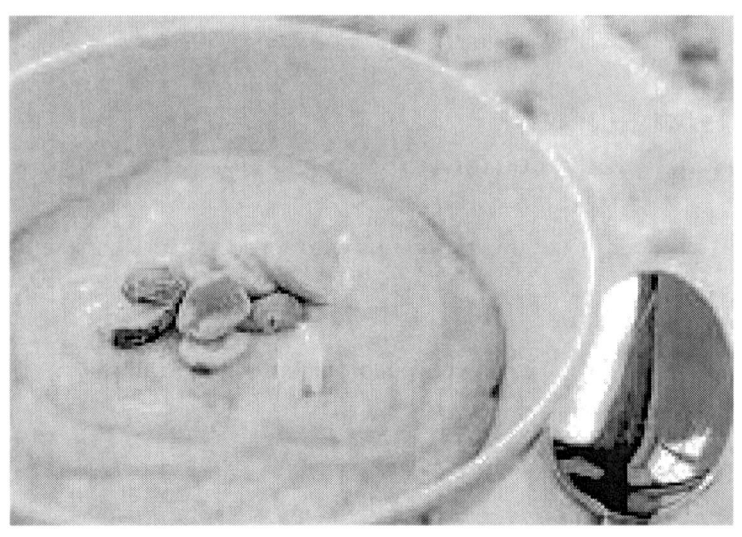

Makes:
8 Servings

Preparation time:
15 minutes

Ingredients:
1/2 cup sugar free peanut butter
3 Tbsp. coconut palm sugar
2 cups coconut milk
2 egg whites
1 tsp. sugarcane juice
1 Tbsp. orange juice
½ tsp. Orange zest

Directions:

1. You can use the blender or an electric mixer for this one. I prefer the electric mixer; it's just easier to clean!

2. In a large bowl, pour the ingredients and mix well.

3. Cover your bowl and refrigerate the pudding for a few hours before you serve it.

Nutrition Information per serving: 217 Calories, 9 g total fat, 91 mg cholesterol, 262 mg sodium, **22 g carbonates (sugars),** 2g fiber, and 11g protein.

SCOTTISH LIKE SCONES

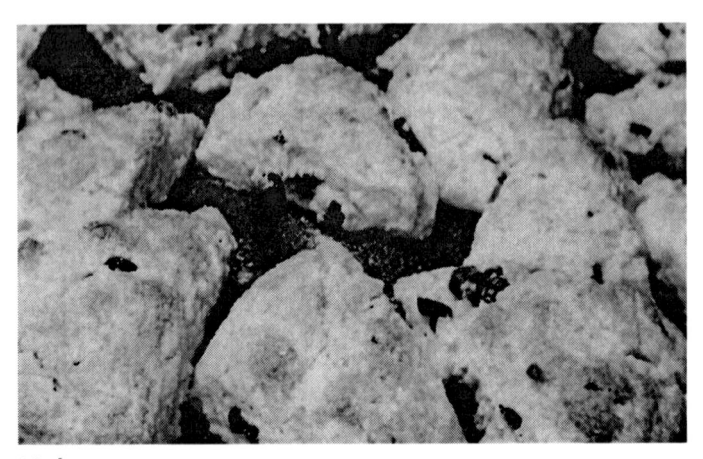

Makes:
16 Servings

Preparation time:
15 minutes

Ingredients:
1 cup quinoa flour
1 cup almond flour
1 tsp. baking powder
1/2 tsp. salt
1 cup fat free sour cream
2 Tbsp. gee butter
½ cup dried raisins
¼ cup dried cherries

Directions:
1. Preheat your oven to 375 degrees F.

2. Prepare a baking sheet by spraying with cooking oil.

3. In a mixing bowl, combine the almond flour, baking powder, salt and quinoa flour.

4. Add the butter, sour cream and mix with your fingers or a fork, your choice.

5. Finally add the dried fruits. Roll the dough until it becomes about ½ inch thick.

6. Cut it into 12-16 pieces to form the scones.

7. Bake on the baking sheet for about 20 minutes.

Nutrition Information per serving: 97 Calories, 3 g total fat, 7 mg cholesterol, 115 mg sodium, **16 g carbonates (sugars),**1.5g fiber, and 3g protein.

FRUITS SKEWERS

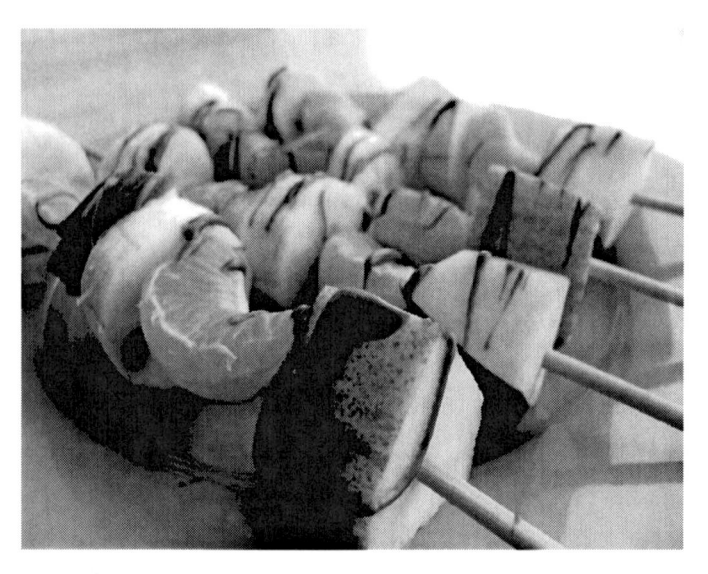

Makes:
4 Servings

Preparation time:
15 minutes

Ingredients:
2 orange peeled and in segments
2 apples (large cubed)
1 banana (thickly sliced)
Any other fruits you would like to include...
2 Tbsp. unsweetened cocoa powder
3 Tbsp. coconut cream
2 Tbsp. coconut palm sugar

Directions:
1. In a small saucepan, mix the coconut milk,, coconut palm sugar and cocoa powder . Bring to boil if needed to get it thick enough so it can act as your chocolate sauce.

2. Arrange all fruits as described.

3. Use wooden skewers and one by one poke through each piece of fruits. Assemble as you wish, no specific order.

4. Drizzle onto each skewer with the chocolate sauce you created.

Nutrition Information per serving: 100 Calories, 1 g total fat, 15 mg cholesterol, 19 mg sodium, **18 g carbonates (sugars),** 1g fiber, and 2g protein.

ORANGE APPLE CLAFOUTI

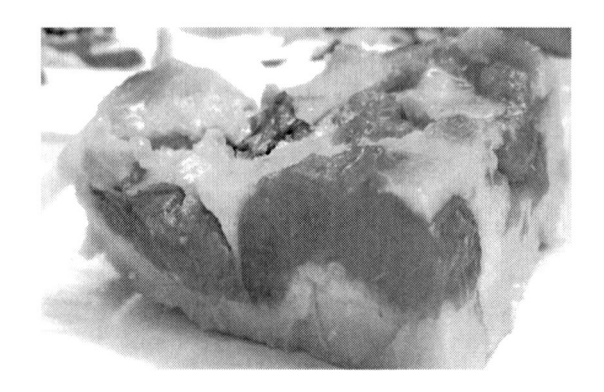

Makes:
8 Servings

Preparation time:
45 minutes

Ingredients:
2-cups of sugar free tangerine or clementine slices with juice (from a can is fine)
1 large diced apple (Gala is great)
2 large eggs
4 egg whites
1/3 cup coconut palm sugar
¾ cups unsweetened coconut milk
1 tsp. vanilla
2 Tbsp. no sugar added orange juice (the juice from the can is fine)
1 Tbsp. orange zest
2/3 cup coconut flour
Pinch salt

Directions:
1. Preheat oven to 375 degrees F.

2. Using the electric mixer, mix the eggs, egg whites and coconut sugar. Next add the coconut milk and, orange juice and vanilla.

3. Finally add the orange zest, coconut flour and combine all together.

4. Use a large baking dish and greased lightly with coconut oil. Place the fruits in the bottom and pour the batter on top.

5. Bake in the oven for 30 minutes.

Nutrition Information per serving: 150 Calories, 2 g total fat, 55 mg cholesterol, 100 mg sodium, **25 g carbonates (sugars),** 1g fiber, and 5g protein.

REINVENTEED ANGEL FOOD CAKE

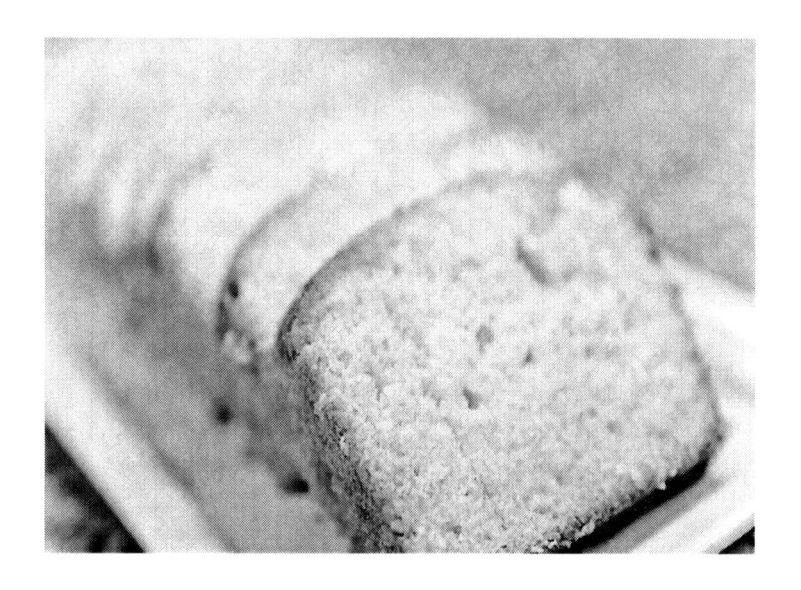

Makes:
10-12 Servings

Preparation time:
50 minutes

Ingredients:

1 cup pure stevia or any equivalent

½ cup non-salted ghee butter

2 large eggs

1 ½ cup coconut flour

1 tsp. baking powder

½ cup unsweetened coconut milk

1 Tbsp. orange zest

Topping

4 Tbsp. orange juice (no sugar added)

1 Tbsp. Sugarcane juice

3 Tbsp. coconut palm sugar

Directions:
1. Preheat oven to 350 degrees F.

2. In a large bowl, whisk well the stevia, butter and eggs. Add all the other ingredients (except the ones for the topping), and combine well.

3. Pour the batter into a greased cake baking dish. Bake for about 50 minutes.

4. Meanwhile, prepare the topping by mixing the 3 ingredient sin a small saucepan. Add on the cake when it just comes out of the oven.

5. Let it cool down 10 minutes after before you start slicing and serving.

Nutrition Information per serving: 157 Calories, 1 g total fat, 20 mg cholesterol, 230 mg sodium, **15 g carbonates (sugars),** 7g fiber, and 4g protein.

CUTE ELEPHANT EARS

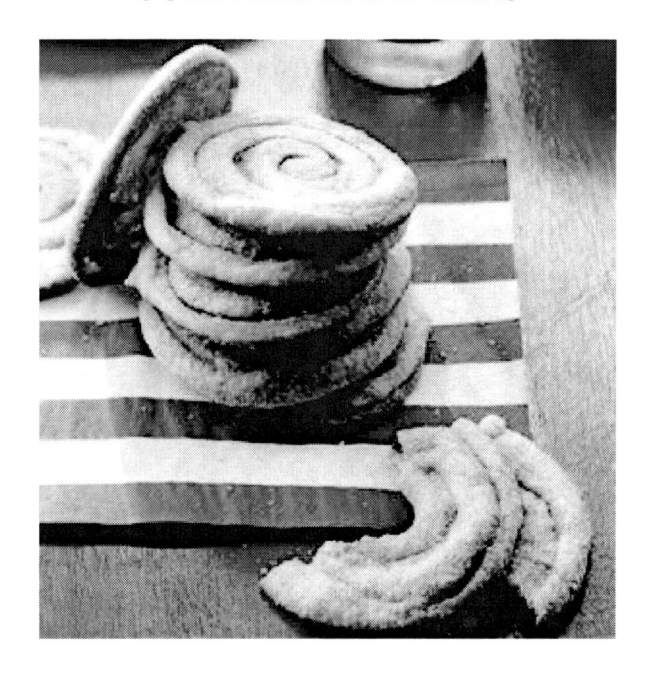

Makes:
24 Servings

Preparation time:
35 minutes

Ingredients:

1 package (1/4 ounce) active dry yeast

1/4 cup warm water

2 cups almond flour

2 Tbsp. pure stevia

Pinch salt

1/3 cup room temperature coconut toil

1/3 cup unsweetened almond milk

1 large egg

Filling

2 Tbsp. coconut oil

1/2 cup coconut palm sugar

1 Tbsp. cinnamon

Directions:

1. Preheat oven to 375 degrees F.

2. In a bowl, ix the dry yeast with warm water and stir until completely dissolved.

3. In a different bowl, mix the almond flour, stevia, salt. Add gradually the coconut oil and you will obtain a crumbly batter.

4. Add next the almond milk, egg. Use your hands next to mix the batter transforming into dough. Cover the bowl with the dough and put in the refrigerator for2 hours.

5. Use a floury surface and roll the dough into a large rectangle.

6. Prepare the filling by mixing all the ingredients in a bowl. Sprinkle the filling on to the dough and roll the dough as you would for a log. Cut the dough into ½ inch slice.

7. Place on slices on a greased baking sheet and cook for about 9-10 minutes. You should obtain about 24 elephant ears total.

Nutrition Information per serving: 109 Calories, 14g total fat, 18 mg cholesterol, 76 mg sodium, **18 g carbonates (sugars),** 0g fiber, and 1g protein.

YOUR DIABETIC EGGNOG VERSION

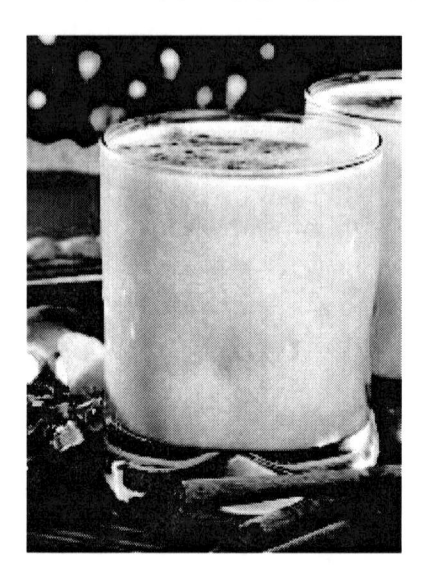

Makes:
4 Servings

Preparation time:
20 minutes

Ingredients:

1 Tbsp. unflavored gelatin

2 cups reduced-fat and sugar free eggnog

2 Tbsp. pure Stevia

¼ tsp. nutmeg

1/2 tsp. almond extract

1 cup sugar free whipped topping, divided

Directions:

1. In a medium saucepan, mix the eggnog and gelatin and let it stand for 5 minutes. Start heating the mix on low temperature and stir in gradually the stevia, nutmeg.

2. When all dissolved, transfer into a bowl and add the almond extract. Refrigerate until ready to serve, in next hour. The eggnog will thicken and that's exactly what you want.

3. Serve with generous portion of whipped cream.

4. You should be able to serve 4 people with this recipe.

Nutrition Information per serving: 165 Calories, 6g total fat, 97 mg cholesterol, 80 mg sodium, **21 g carbonates (sugars),** 1g fiber, and 7g protein.

STRAWBERRY PARFAIT

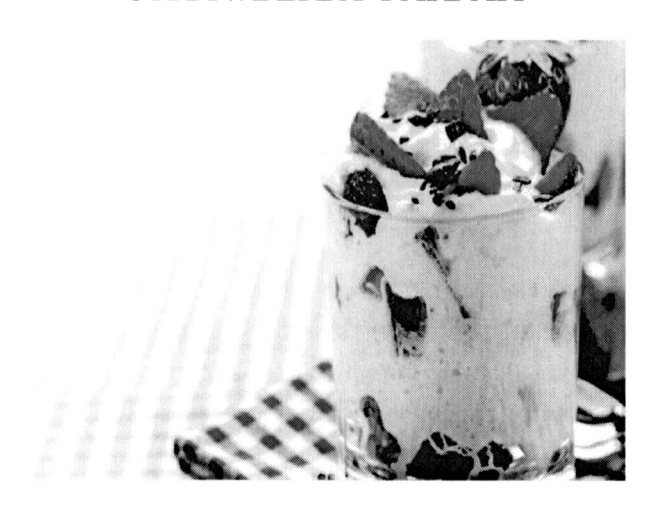

Makes:
2-4 Servings

Preparation time:
30 minutes

Ingredients:
1 small sugar free pack strawberry gelatin (Jello)

1 cup boiling water

2 egg whites

1 cup fresh sliced strawberry

½ cup fresh blueberries

1 Tbsp. chia seeds

1 Tbsp. orange zest

Directions:
1. Dissolve the strawberry gelatin in the boiling water and then cool as instructed on the package. Add the egg whites.

2. Use an electric mixer and mix the *jello* with the egg whites for 6 or 7 minutes.

3. Add the strawberries, blue berries, and orange zest and chia seeds. Mix again.

4. Pour the final mixture into fancy cups.

Nutrition Information per serving: 61 Calories, 14g total fat, 0 mg cholesterol, 56 mg sodium, **13 g carbonates (sugars),** 1g fiber, and 3g protein.

DELICIOUS BANANA AND MORE COOKIES

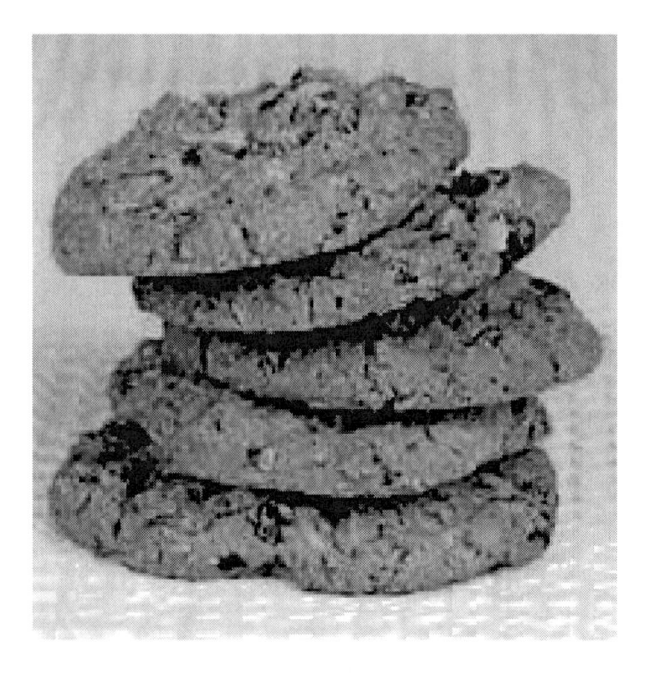

Makes:
30 Servings

Preparation time:
30 minutes

Ingredients:
1.5 cups quinoa flour

½ cup flaxseeds

1 tsp. baking powder

½ tsp. baking soda

1 tsp. cinnamon

1 tsp. vanilla

Pinch salt

2 large ripe bananas

2 Tbsp. coconut oil

¾ cup coconut palm sugar

3/4 cup chopped walnuts

2 Tbsp., Manuka honey

Directions:
1. Preheat oven to 350 degrees F.

2. Spray nonstick cooking spray on 2 large baking sheets.

3. In a mixing bowl, mash the bananas; add the eggs, vanilla, coconut oil and honey.

4. In a larger bowl, mix the dry ingredients: quinoa flour, flaxseeds, coconut palm sugar, baking soda, baking powder, cinnamon and salt.

5. Combine the wet mixture into the dry well and mix well.

6. Add the walnuts and mix again. Drop a teaspoon of cookie dough at a time on the baking sheets and you should be able to make about 24-30 servings.

7. Bake for 15 minutes or so, watch closely.

Nutrition Information per serving: 80 Calories, 3g total fat, 5 mg cholesterol, 35 mg sodium, **11.5 g carbonates (sugars),** 1.5g fiber, and 2g protein.

A DIABETIC GREEN TEA SMOOTHIE

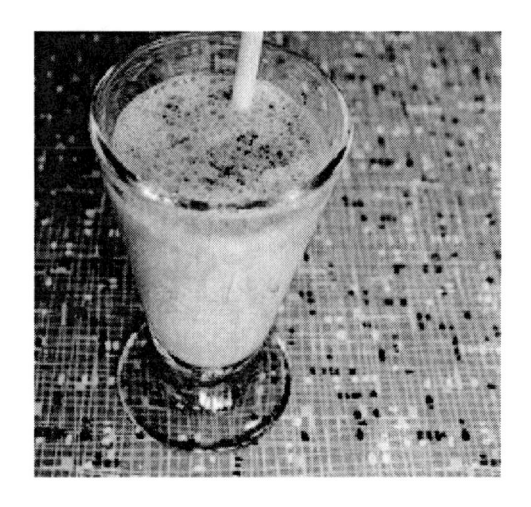

Makes:
1 serving

Preparation time:
10 minutes

Ingredients:

2 Tbsp. sugar free green tea powder

3 Tbsp. hot water

1 banana

1 cup almond milk

½ cup ice cubed

1 Tbsp. Manuka honey

Directions:

1. In a bowl, mix the green tea and water together. Blend all the ingredients, including the green teat paste together in your high speed blender.

2. Add more ice cubes if you wish.

Nutrition Information per serving: 95 Calories, 1g total fat, 0 mg cholesterol, 35 mg sodium, **16.5 g carbonates (sugars),** 1.5g fiber, and 2g protein.

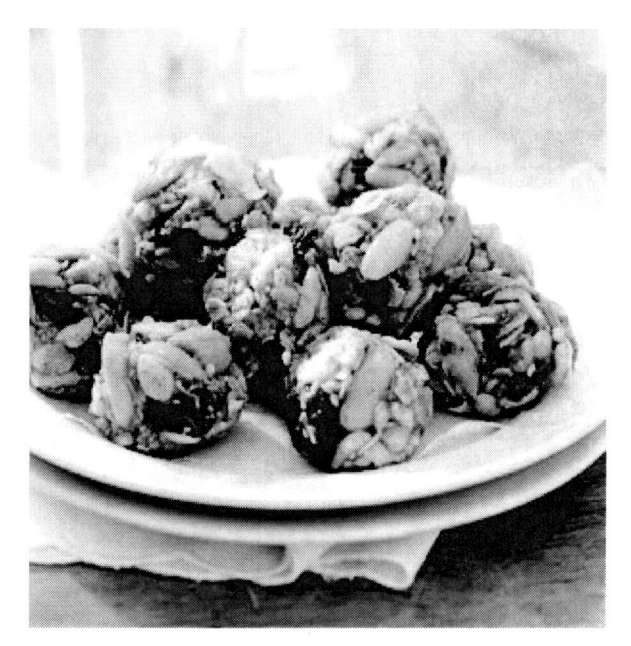

SOME BALLS OF GOODNESS

Makes:
24-30 servings

Preparation time:
1.5 hour

Ingredients:
1/3 cup Manuka honey
2 Tbsp. orange juice (no sugar added)
½ cup almond butter
¼ cup flaxseeds
½ cup coconut flour
1/3 dried cranberries
¼ cup chopped cashews

1/4 cup unsweetened flaked coconut
1 Tbsp. sesame seeds

Directions:
1. In a small saucepan, mix in the orange juice and honey and heat on low temperature. Remove from heat.

2. Add the almond butter with the honey mixture, and mix until the mixture becomes smooth.

3. In a large mixing bowl, combine next the flaxseeds, coconut flour, cashews, cranberries, coconut flakes and sesame seeds.

4. Next step is to pour the honey and almond butter on top of the dry ingredients. Cover the bowl and refrigerate for about 1 hour.

5. When you take the mixture out, it should be just right to mold into balls. You should be able to form about 24-20 balls total.

Nutrition Information per serving: 153 Calories, 8g total fat, 100 mg cholesterol, 48 mg sodium, **17 g carbonates (sugars),** 2g fiber, and 4g protein.

YUMMY SANDWICH COOKIES

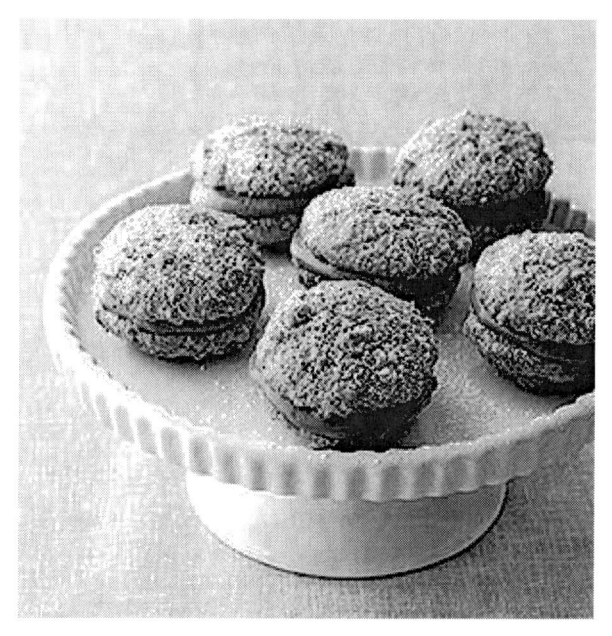

Makes:
24 servings

Preparation time:
10 minutes

Ingredients:
½ cup coconut flour
1 tsp. baking powder
5 eggs
2/3 cup coconut palm sugar
2 cup toasted pecans
½ cup fat free cream cheese
2 Tbsp. unsweetened cocoa powder
2 Tbsp. skim milk

Directions:

1. Preheat oven to 350 degrees F.

2. Combine in large bowl the coconut flour, baking powder and mix well.

3. In the food processor, mix the eggs, coconut palm sugar and nuts and activate until it is almost smooth. Add this new mixture to their first flour one.

4. You now have your cookie dough and form the cookies and place them on a previously greased baking sheet a few inches apart. Bake for 10 minutes.

5. When they come out, let them cool down some and then mix together in a small bowl what will be the filling: cream cheese, milk and cocoa powder.

6. Fill each cookie with about a teaspoon of chocolate mixture (like a sandwich, a cookie on the bottom and one of the top).

Nutrition Information per serving: 92 Calories, 4.5g total fat, 10 mg cholesterol, 109 mg sodium, **10 g carbonates (sugars),** 1g fiber, and 3g protein.

THIS MAGESTIC BANANAS AND BERRIES TREAT

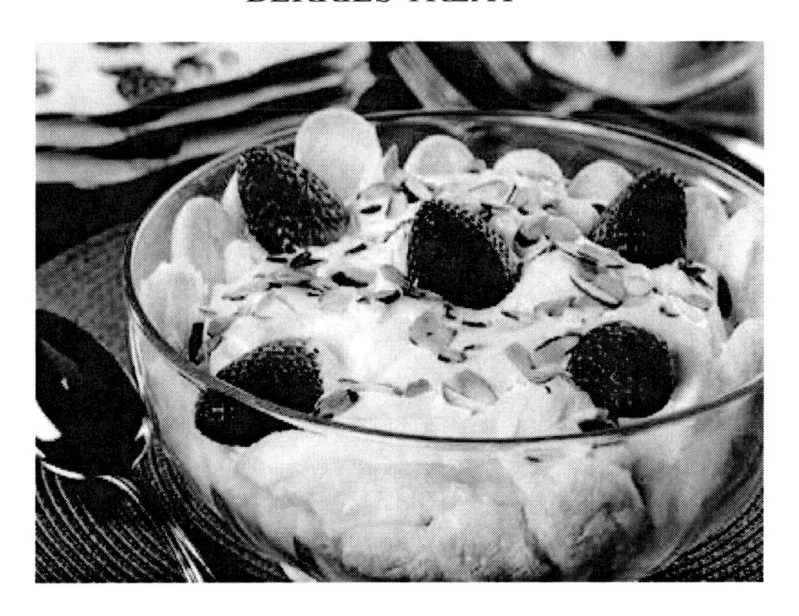

Makes:
12 servings

Preparation time:
25 minutes

Ingredients:
1 package of sugar free vanilla pudding mix
2 tsp. vanilla extract
2 cups unsweetened coconut milk
1 cup sliced fresh strawberries
1 or 2 sliced bananas
2 Tbsp. pure Stevia

3 Tbsp. favorite nuts (I prefer chopped pecans)

Directions:
1. First, prepare the pudding according to the directions on the package, using the coconut milk. Place in the refrigerator for now.

2. In a small bowl, place the fresh strawberries with the Stevia and vanilla and mix well.

3. Remove the pudding from the refrigerator, make sure it is place in your serving bowl, and let's assemble.

4. Place the sliced bananas around the pudding evenly and the strawberries so it looks pretty.

5. Sprinkle the nuts on top and serve cold.

Nutrition Information per serving: 196 Calories, 2.5g total fat, 25 mg cholesterol, 109 mg sodium, **22 g carbonates (sugars),** 2g fiber, and 3g protein.

CHOCO-CHEESE NO BAKE PIE

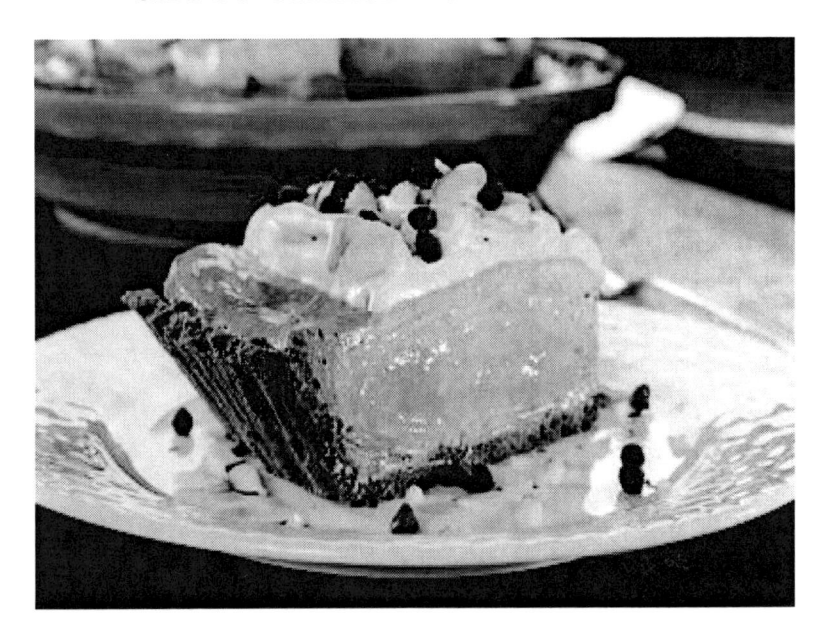

Makes:
8 servings

Preparation time:
35 minutes

Ingredients:
2 fat free packages cream cheese (room temperature)
1 package sugar free chocolate pudding mix
1 cup unsweetened almond milk
¼ cup water
1 tsp. almond extract

1 cup sugar free whipped cream

Pie crust:
I highly suggest you purchase a sugar free chocolate cookie crust to make your life easier

Directions:

1. First, in a large bowl, combine the cream cheese, the almond milk and the chocolate pudding mix, and water. Mix very well.

2. Combine the almond extract and also the whipped cream to the first mixture. Mix again.

3. Spread the pie filling on the pre-cooked crust evenly.

4. You can decorate with nuts, carob chips, or just eat it as is, because it is definitely very smooth and tasty.

Nutrition Information per serving: 202 Calories, 4.5g total fat, 23 mg cholesterol, 100 mg sodium, **25 g carbonates (sugars),** 1g fiber, and 3g protein.

CHOCOLATE MINTY PUDDING

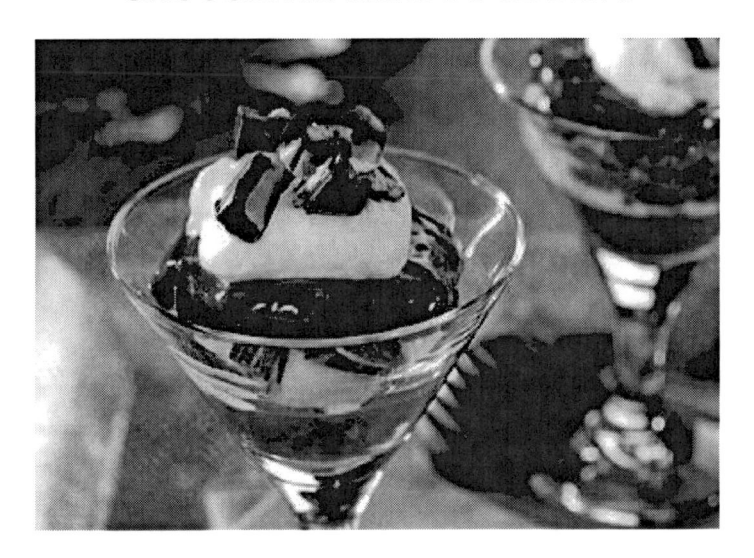

Makes:
4-6 serving

Preparation time:
30 minutes

Ingredients:
 1 package of sugar free chocolate pudding mix
 3 tbsp. crushed sugar free peppermints
 2 cups unsweetened cashew milk
 ½ cup sugar free whipped cream

Directions:

1. Prepare pudding according to package directions, using the cashew milk. Refrigerate for at least 15 minutes.

2. Meanwhile use a food processor to crush the mints so they are as small as possible.

3. Remove the pudding from the refrigerator; add the whipped cream and the crushed candies. Separate in serving bowls, and enjoy!

Nutrition Information per serving: 143 Calories, 2.5g total fat, 12 mg cholesterol, 100 mg sodium, **15 g carbonates (sugars),** 1.5g fiber, and 2g protein.

AVOCADO AND PEANUT BUTTER SHAKE

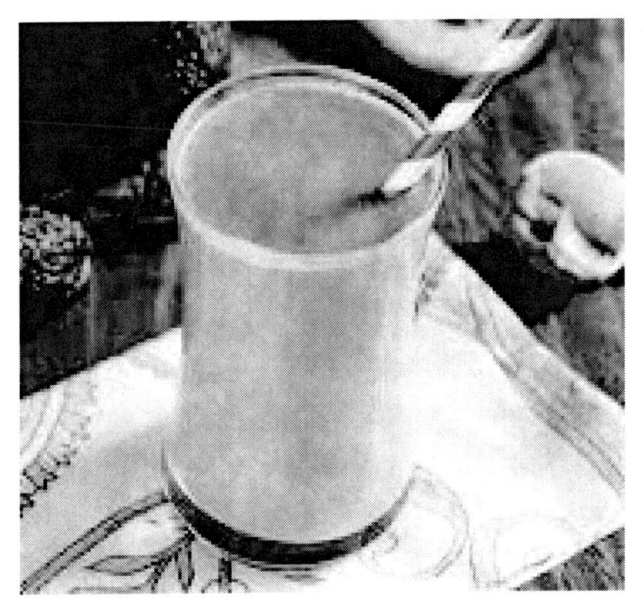

Makes:
1 serving

Preparation time:
10 minutes

Ingredients:
½ ripe avocado
2 Tbsp. creamy sugar free peanut butter
1 tsp. lemon juice
1 cup unsweetened cashew milk
1 cup ice cubes

Directions:

1. Easy enough. Blend all the ingredients in the high speed blender.

2. If the shake would become too thick, add more ice cubes and mix again.

3. When you are happy with the texture, pour into your tallest cup. Enjoy …

Nutrition Information per serving: 159 Calories, 2.9g total fat, 98 mg cholesterol, 109 mg sodium, **16 g carbonates (sugars),** 1g fiber, and 3g protein.

PINEAPPLE SIMPLE BARS

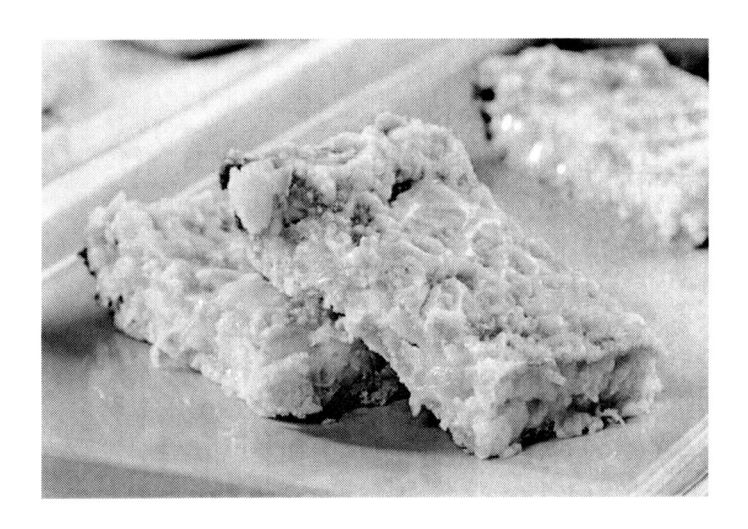

Makes:
10-12 servings

Preparation time:
1 hour

Ingredients:
Crust
1 ½ cup coconut flour
¼ cup coconut palm sugar
Pinch salt
¼ cup coconut oil (room temperature)
Filling
2 large eggs
½ cup fat free sour cream
1/3 cup coconut flour
1 can sugar free crushed pineapple (drained)
Topping (drizzle)

2 Tbsp. coconut milk
1/3 cup coconut palm sugar

Directions:
1. Preheat oven to 350 degrees F.
2. In a mixing bowl, to prepare the crust, mix all the ingredients. Press into a greased rectangle baking dish and bake in the oven for about 20 minutes.
3. In a different bowl, combine the eggs, sour cream and coconut flour. Add gradually the crushed pineapple and stir well. Spread this mixture on the cooled down crust evenly.
4. Place again in the oven for another 45 to 50 minutes.
5. Meanwhile, mix together the topping ingredients. When the dessert is cooked, you can choose to drizzle over it and cut into bars to serve.

Nutrition Information per serving: 159 Calories, 2.9g total fat, 98 mg cholesterol, 109 mg sodium, **16 g carbonates (sugars),** 1g fiber, and 3g protein.